KNOW THE ENEMY

PREVENTING WEIGHT GAIN, DIABETES, & DISEASE

By Jodi Velazquez

Copyright 2024

Jodi Velazquez

This book was produced and printed in the United States of America

Proprietary Notice

All Rights Reserved. No part of this book may be reproduced in whole or in part without written permission form the publisher, except by reviewers who may quote brief excerpts in connection with a book review in a newspaper, magazine, or electronic publication, nor may any part of this book be reproduced, stored in a retrieval system, or transmitted in any form or by any means electronic, mechanical, photocopying, recording, or other, without written permission from the publisher.

Release Date 2024

Published by Atlas Elite Publishing

ISBN 979-8-9915524-1-7

Slick Move, LLC

P.O. Box 243

Presto, PA 15142

Get in touch with the author

Website: http://www.jodivelazquez.com/

Facebook: https://www.facebook.com/jodi.velazquez.5

Instagram: jodivelazquez

Order this book in bulk:

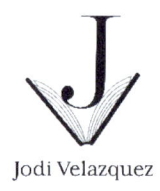

Jodi Velazquez

slickmoveguide@comcast.net

Disclaimer

This book is a memoir. It contains the recollection and thoughts of the author. This book is not intended to replace the services of a physician or dietician. Any application of the recommendations set forth in the following pages is at the reader's discretion. Individuals are advised to consult with his or her physician, dietician, or appropriate health care professional before undertaking any dietary or exercise recommendations in this publication. If you or someone you are caring for are under medical guidance/treatment consult with a physician before making any changes in the medical regiment. Professionals must use and apply their own judgment, experience, and training and should not rely solely on the information contained in this publication. The author assumes no responsibility or liability for personal or other injury, loss, or damage that may result from the suggestions or information in this publication.

All claims expressed in this article are solely those of the authors and do not necessarily represent those of their affiliated organizations, or those of the publisher, the editors, and the reviewers. Any product that may be evaluated in this article, or claim that may be made by its manufacturer, is not guaranteed, or endorsed by the publisher. Reasonable steps have been taken to ensure the accuracy of the information and research presented. The materials and information in this publication are intended for informational purposes only. Some of the information may be dated and may not reflect the most current developments. The views, thoughts, and opinions expressed in the text belong solely to the author, and not necessarily to the author's employer, organization, committee, or other group or individual.

Acknowledgments and Sincere thanks to:

Editing – Medical Journal Editors https://www.medicaljournaleditors.com
Contributor – Theresa Ivancik https://theresaivancik.com/
Cover Design – Michael Beas
Formatting – Tom Colleran
Logo Design – Nicole Suchin www.nicolesuchin.com
Preliminary Proofreading and Fact-Checking – Sean Armstrong
Pre-publication read – Esra Karslioglu French, MD Endocrinology
Pre-publication read – Kathy Harrison, Anna Carlile
Photography – Rene' Michele Photography, LLC
www.renemichelephotographyllc.com
My Mom and Dad

I am so grateful for the super talented and wonderful team at Elite Atlas Publishing Partners for believing in me, being so patient and helping me in so many ways.

Sincere gratitude and thanks for the financial support for this project from:

John Velazquez
Xtreme Car & Truck Accessories
Nicole Radulovich
Brand pH LLC
Robin & Brian Shorr
Joanna Abel
Jeff Moran
Alan & Peggy Ballo
Mari & Jon Grant Family
Chris Vargas
Ian Gallagher
Tara Lee Obrien, author of "Jackpot Junkie"
Annie Budzik

Book Review by Esra Karslioglu French MD, Board certified physician in Endocrinology and Obesity Medicine:

"Numbers are scary: 40% of US population is obese. If you add up overweight people to this number, this makes 70% of our population. Obesity is not an American problem. More than 1 billion people in the world are now living with obesity.

Obesity is the disease of century: it is an end product of our environment. It is almost like fate unless we find a way to break out of this routine lifestyle built for us. Watch more tv, work long hours, eat what is easily available and to relax, watch more tv. It is difficult, we individuals need to fight against our `environment` daily, it can be exhausting.

Thus, we need easy, practical solutions. That`s why Jodi`s book is here to help you. She is a busy working mom, who brought up a kid with Type 1 DM. Over years, she worked with physicians, dietitians, diabetes educators and created a lifestyle to keep her family healthy. She is now sharing her wisdom with all of us. The tips she shared here have a different melody: they are not from an authoritarian health care professional or from theoretical diet books, but from a practical mother who brought up a healthy child with Type 1 DM.

As an endocrinologist, my passion is to keep my patients with diabetes and weight problems healthy. I find in my daily practice, a big void for practical information. We all say to our patients to work out 150 minutes a week. In her book Jodi is showing how she keeps moving while also preparing breakfast for her kids early in the morning before she goes to work. She shows you how and makes it easy for you.

I applaud Jodi`s work and practical wisdom. You can use this book to navigate busy daily life and still win with healthy habits. I will recommend Jodi`s book to all my patients who desires to lose weight and or have a healthy life style. This book bundled with advice from your healthcare professionals will do wonders for you.

It is difficult to lose and maintain a healthy weight but Jodi shows us, it is doable. As Henry Ford said: `whether you think you can, or you think you can't; you're right!`"

Esra Karslioglu *French MD*

Board certified physician in Endocrinology and Obesity Medicine

DEDICATION

I would like to thank my daughter Marlo because without her my eyes never would have been opened to the abundance of knowledge contained in this book about diet and wellness. It has been an honor to help you.

I would like to thank both Marlo and Lanah for their endless support and encouragement during the writing of this book. I am blessed to have you both.

Contents

INTRODUCTION ... 9

CHAPTER 1 ... 13
My Personal Experience

CHAPTER 2 ... 18
Insider Information: Are You Struggling and Want to Know Why?

CHAPTER 3 ... 21
Observation – For Those with Diabetes AND Those Without Diabetes

CHAPTER 4 ... 25
Eliminate Unhealthy Self-Image Thinking

CHAPTER 5 ... 30
Four Key Concepts – ABCTs

CHAPTER 6 ... 33
Roadblocks to the Four Key Concepts-ABCTs

CHAPTER 7 ... 36
Fast Food – What You May Not Know

CHAPTER 8 ... 48
Shocking: Portion Increase

CHAPTER 9 ... 60
Explosion of Food Processing and Packaged Food

CHAPTER 10 ... 70
The Temptation of Time and Convenience

CHAPTER 11 ... 75
Are Food Additives Making Us Fat?

CHAPTER 12 ... 87
Be Smarter – Complex and Simple Carbohydrates

CHAPTER 13 ... 89
High Sugar in Food, Unhealthy High Fat – a Deadly Combination

CHAPTER 14 113
Treats in Schools (Parents Don't Skip This Chapter!)

CHAPTER 15 128
Balance Food and Activity – A Must Know!

CHAPTER 16 131
The Easiest Step – Pack Your Lunch

CHAPTER 17 135
Learn to Flip It—The Most Important Tip in This Book

CHAPTER 18 145
Why Try to Prevent Obesity—What You May Not Know

CHAPTER 19 152
Why Aren't You Exercising? Exercise and Physical Activity

CHAPTER 20 159
Post-Organized Sports

CHAPTER 21 169
What To Look for In a Workout App

CHAPTER 22 176
Injury/Health Issues and Exercise

CHAPTER 23 185
45 Super-Fun Non-Technology Activities for Kids

CONCLUSION – A LIFESTYLE CHANGE 223
ABOUT THE AUTHOR 224

Introduction

Are you trying to decide if you should read this book?

If you are overweight or gaining weight and you are not happy about it, please read this introduction. You may have been told by a doctor, a family member, or a friend that you should lose weight, but you have not been able to. Sometimes learning *why* you should can be helpful. Have you ever said, "I wish I'd known"?

It took me a long time to write this book; I could not figure out why for some time. I had so much information compiled into chapters, but I was struggling. I had a vision and, of course, with most visions, there can be some difficulty in turning them into reality. That is why I wanted to write a book that both overweight people and people with diabetes could read.

My assumption was that a person who was trying to get their weight under control would open this book and see the word "diabetes" or information on diabetes and think, oh this book is not for me, I do not have diabetes.

Today, we live in a world where exposing the truth can be hurtful and/or cause anxiety. We must be careful not to say too much. But wouldn't it make an impact if we could inform people, in detail, so we avoid the negative event occurring in the first place? Doesn't everybody want to avoid negative events?

For example, if you wanted to keep your teenage child from participating in criminal activity, you could schedule a field trip for them to visit a penitentiary, so they can get an idea, a visual one, of where that lifestyle might lead. If a teenager could visit a drug rehab center or emphysema unit in a hospital to see where smoking and drug activity can lead, would this help their decision?

While what you just read may have your mouth dropping, you also may be wondering, would it make a difference? I remember as a teenager seeing a movie called *Midnight Express*. It's about a man who was traveling abroad with drugs and got caught by airport security; he was then put in an overseas prison. Personally, the movie left a lifelong impact on me about the seriousness of drugs. The problem is, sometimes we have trouble differentiating between "movies" and "reality" when at the movie theater. I was fortunate that I saw the movie as a serious possible reality for offenders.

I am a firm believer in teaching with explanation. When I tell my kids that they should not do something, I like to also explain *why* they should not and provide as much detail as possible.

This book is going to suggest how to improve your diet to control your weight. It will also tell you about diabetes, how the foods that you eat, and your lifestyle may play a big part in you avoiding insulin dependency. By learning a little about diabetes while reading about a healthy diet, you will increase your chances of preventing it.

If you are overweight and you refuse to read this book because it talks about diabetes, then you are refusing to get on the field trip bus. Believe me, the positive and helpful dietary information you will learn from reading this book will far outweigh the difficulty of reading a little about diabetes.

Read this book and you will understand how to maintain a better diet and possibly avoid diabetes. Be in the know before it is too late.

What is the enemy? The variety of contributing factors that have created the current obesity epidemic in the United States – what this book is all about! From a wellness standpoint, it became my mission to know what was bad for my family and learn what could keep us healthy. Understanding the enemy is the key to winning the battle!

> If you know the enemy and know yourself, you need not fear the result of a hundred battles. If you know yourself, but not the enemy, for every victory gained you will also suffer a defeat. If you know neither, the enemy nor yourself, you will succumb in every battle.
>
> - Sun Tzu, ancient Chinese warrior

There is Proof: Diabetes and Obesity Work Hand-in-Hand

Of the people diagnosed with Type 2 diabetes, 89% percent are also diagnosed as overweight or obese.[1] This fact provides an interesting clue to the link between diabetes and obesity. Being overweight places extra stress on your body in a variety of ways, including your body's ability to maintain proper blood glucose levels. In fact, being overweight can cause your body to become resistant to insulin. If you already have diabetes, this means you will need to take even more insulin to get sugar into your cells. And if you don't have diabetes, the prolonged effects of insulin resistance can eventually cause you to develop the disease.

To reduce the chances that you will develop diabetes it is helpful to maintain a healthy weight and increase your physical activity. If you are overweight, even a small weight loss (5 to 10 percent) can prevent diabetes[2]—or prolong the chance that you will develop the disease—even if you fall into a high-risk category.

Who Will This Book Help?

• This book will benefit anyone who wants to improve their overall diet and health by becoming aware of the factors in our society that make it hard for us to eat healthy and stay fit.

• If you or your child are overweight and desire to lose weight to get on the road to a healthier lifestyle, this book is for you.

• If you have trouble understanding why it is so hard for you to lose weight and/or control your diabetes, this book will explain "the why."

• If you are overweight and worried about getting Type 2, then this book will help you.

• If you have Type 2 diabetes and are treating it with pills or if you want to keep your blood sugar in a good range to avoid becoming dependent on insulin, then this book can be a great help to you.

• If you have Type 1 diabetes or have a child or loved one with diabetes, you will benefit from reading this book.

• If you are a caretaker, grandparent, daycare attendant, or teacher and you want to create a healthy environment for those in your care, then this book is for you.

Are You Ready for a Positive Change? Take It Slow.

To make changes in life, it is necessary to look at our history to understand why we need to change. The United States, currently, has a problem with obesity and diabetes not only among adults and the elderly, but children too. According to the United States Centers for Disease Control and Prevention, 34.2 million people, or 10.5% of the American population, have diabetes. As many as 88 million adult Americans (18 and older) have prediabetes, which is about 34.5 percent of the population.[1] In this book, I will look at the past and compare it to the present to reveal reasons for this problem. While it would be nice if there was a single solution, unfortunately, there are a variety of factors that have contributed to obesity and diabetes in the United States. I will talk about some circumstances that you may not even be aware of that may affect you and or your ability to lose weight and control diabetes, as well as what you can do about it. Trying to change too much at one time will probably overwhelm you. Take it slow and, little by little, your changes will all add up. Habits are hard to change, so your desire is going to have to be strong. Start believing that you are strong, and you will make changes that will improve and, possibly, save your life. The advice in this book is attainable.

Literature Cited in this Chapter

1. National Diabetes Statistics Report. United States Centers for Disease Prevention and Control. January 28, 2024. https://www.cdc.gov/diabetes/php/data-research/?CDC_AAref_Val=https://www.cdc.gov/diabetes/data/statistics-report/index.html

2. Diabetes Prevention: 5 Tips for Taking Control. Mayo Clinic. March 24, 2023. https://www.mayoclinic.org/diseases-conditions/type-2-diabetes/in-depth/diabetes-prevention/art-20047639

Chapter 1

My Personal Experience

The sole purpose of this book is to use my personal experience to provide advice, ideas, and support to enhance people's health by making better food and lifestyle choices. We all desire to be healthy and fit, but what makes it easier for some than others? Many have given in and are saying, "It is genetic, this is the way that I am built." But are you willing to just accept that? After you read this book you may understand, a little better, how many factors in our society are teaming up against you to make it hard for you to eat healthily and maintain a good weight. **Once you realize how much the enemy has infiltrated your everyday environment, you may understand a little better why you are having so much trouble. The opponent has surrounded you, but I am going to tell you how to become a "Green Beret" who can slip through the traps, to get on the road to better health and fitness.**

You may be wondering what the difference is between this book and all the other food and diet books. That answer lies in my personal experience. My first daughter was diagnosed at just 19 months old with Type 1 diabetes. When you are diagnosed with diabetes, you or your parents are informed that you must eat right to maintain a good blood sugar level. Initially, very little education tends to be provided to help you accomplish this difficult task. Furthermore, what many people do not realize is once you are diagnosed, you are required to report back to the doctor every three months and have a blood test to check your A1C.

An A1C test measures a person's average blood glucose levels over the past two to three months and that number will show how well you did for that period. That's right: how well you did or didn't do will be exposed. If you do not like being monitored, you may not like this. If you do a good job and your blood sugar A1C is in a good range (less than 7 is desired), you get the thumbs up. Sometimes small children are permitted to have a higher A1C to avoid hypoglycemic events or dangerously low blood sugar. If it is not in a good range, then your doctor will most likely remind you of the dangers of high blood sugar and want to work with you to make changes, including an effort to lower the blood sugar through diet, exercise, and insulin adjustments.

Since my daughter was only 19 months old when she was diagnosed, I had to learn for her about how to maintain a good blood sugar level through food and lifestyle. Since she was barely a toddler, it was recommended that she test her blood sugar 10 times a day to avoid it dropping too low. She did not understand that she should tell me when she felt poorly, and that was the reason for the close observation. **With such close monitoring, I could see how every kind of food affected her blood sugar and what certain activities, specific exercises, and being sedentary did to her blood sugar. I have witnessed first-hand through daily blood sugar numbers what the challenges of a healthy American diet are all about. These challenges are not just food challenges.** I am officially a "Green Beret" successfully battling the poor "American Diet" and you can be a "Green Beret" too!

While I am not professionally educated in the field of childhood development or health care, it is my experience as well as my dedication and continuous effort to keep my daughter in good health, that gives me the knowledge to speak on this subject. Up until she became an adult, my daughter had never had an A1C over 7.4. Due to the events, conditions, and circumstances that I encountered daily for over a decade and a half, I believe that I can offer extraordinary insight to people, parents, and caretakers who want to improve their health and lifestyle—or the health and lifestyle of their loved ones. I believe that because of my necessary close observation, monitoring, and involvement, I can advise with factual proof on several issues that are health- and welfare-related.

The Beat Begins and My Initial Observations

In 1999, many were concerned about Y2K: the world was supposed to stop as computers encountered the turn of the century. This was a time when computer programmers feared programs would not interpret 00 as 2000. All computers were expected to have malfunctioned, and the world would experience extensive havoc. I had some sort of women's intuition going on, so I thought. I was living in New York and decided to get on a plane, days before that dreaded New Year's Eve, to be with my parents in Pennsylvania. At least my newborn baby and I would be out of the big city where total chaos could break out. Then the clock hit midnight—and nothing. However, the real disaster that I think my intuition had picked up on happened 11 months later, on December 11, 2000, when my 19-month-old daughter was diagnosed with Type 1 diabetes. That was earth-shaking for me. During that time, I had just found out that I was pregnant with my second child. I was not prepared for all of this; but, as many mothers do, I mustered up the strength and got right to work doing what I had to do to make sure my daughter would live as healthy a life as she could.

For over 16 years, my daughter and I worked together to do the hourly job of her non-active pancreas: making sure that her blood sugar numbers stayed within a good range. When she was a toddler, I would make decisions every two hours about what she should eat, and how much; and what to do if her blood sugar was high or low. Once in school, she followed the chart that I made for her, so she could make the needed adjustments herself to stay in range. We had great control working as a team throughout the years. After 18 or so, she started managing her condition completely on her own. I wanted to put forth my best effort to preserve her health during her younger years by keeping her blood sugar in a good range for her. Hopefully, she will continue the beat of striving for good health through college, getting married, or any other stage in her life.

A Reason for Exercise and Creative Play – Put in the Effort to Get Moving

Having an infant with insulin-dependent diabetes posed a few challenges. After many sleepless nights due to finger checks as well as unstable blood sugar levels, my husband and I became very tired. At such a young age, my daughter was not able to express her feelings about how she felt, so we did plenty of guessing and worrying. Since we did not have many people who offered to take our kids for the day, we did not get breaks often.

We weren't participating in daily exercise and our stress levels were reaching heights that were unsafe. After a couple of years went by, I was able to stop thinking so much about my daughter's health and I began to realize that my accelerated adrenaline level would eventually take me down if I continued at the pace I was going. My daughter was approaching 4 years old and able to sit and watch TV or color for hours. Ahhhh, this was nice. I noticed that her blood sugar did not drop so much when she sat still for a long time, unlike the years prior, where she seemed to always be running, which kept us mostly dealing with low blood sugar. Now that she was calmer, we were seeing a change in the averages. They were getting higher. Argh! This was bad. We realized that we had a serious need for daily exercise to keep blood sugar balanced; we could not just put her in front of the TV all the time.

That is when our need for exercise and "creative play" began. After a finger check that showed a blood sugar number on the higher side, my husband and I would say, "Let's get her moving." The idea was that getting active would not only benefit my daughter's blood sugar but our health as well. Our second daughter, who was a newborn, was also getting a lot of action with all the playing, so she was sleeping very well at night, which was a real bonus. It was easy in the summer, but in the winter months, we had to get creative. Our house became a unique play area. We had to give up on society's rules of the perfectly neat household. When our kids' friends would come over to play, they couldn't believe some stuff that we were doing! At the end of this book, I will share many of our favorite creative play games for our kids that got them moving and helped keep their blood sugar in a good range. Any amount of movement helps decrease blood sugar. Rule number one for us was to **Get Moving!** A sedentary lifestyle does not burn calories or bring down blood sugar!

More Reasons for Creative Play – Mental Benefit

Although we will never know why or how my daughter developed diabetes as a baby, there is always a part of me that has felt that maybe it was something that I may have done to cause it. Having your finger pricked 10 times a day and two or three insulin injections would be tough. My heart breaks, even now, when I think about it. She is in her twenties and hardly ever complains. This is another reason why I always made an extra effort to try to make her days fun through creative play and games when she was young. I just wanted to see her smiling and laughing. I have enjoyed giving both of my daughters a lot of attention by playing fun games with them. Once, my daughter brought a Mother's Day card home from school that she made for me. She sat next to me as I read the card and it said, "What I like about my Mom: I like when she buys me new toys and clothes, I like when she cooks good food for me and when she cleans my room. But what I especially like is when she plays with me."

Kids just want your time. If you are too overwhelmed to think of a game to play or something to do with your child, then you have hit the wall! Slide down off the wall, stand up, and shake it off; They are only young for a very short time; in just the blink of an eye, they will be big! Take a deep breath, put on some comfortable clothes, put away the cell phone and electronics, forget about what needs to be done, and start playing. Plus, the activities can surely take your mind off anything that is bothering you. Putting in time with your children is always positive and it makes you feel good inside. Plus, you make your kids smile and laugh when you play with them. Remember this: stress can raise blood sugar, and laughter can reduce blood sugar. You will benefit, both physically and mentally, which can, in turn, improve your health! So not only did we have to watch what kinds of foods we were eating, but we had to also incorporate activity. Put a limit on your laptop, phone, electronic game time, or whatever your sedentary crutch might be so you can get your body moving.

CHAPTER 2

Insider Information: Are You Struggling and Want to Know Why?

You may feel as if you are bombarded with way too much information about diets. They can range from the Keto diet to the Paleo diet or even never eating meat or dairy again. It is confusing and may sometimes leave you wondering *what the best diet is.* You may have tried diets and been initially successful, only to quit shortly after and regain all the weight you have lost. You may have given up and are speaking out about being proud of your size, but, in the meantime, your doctor is warning you and you feel awful. You may look at thin and fit people and wonder what they are doing that is so different from what you are doing. I'm going to tell you: it's not one thing, it is many things. And, once I point them all out to you, the picture will be much clearer than a crystal ball. Just like diabetes, weight control is hard to understand, and it is not your fault if you have been unsuccessful. You are basically trying to achieve the same goal as **someone with diabetes which is to eat healthily; but you need this to become your lifestyle.** While I am sure that you have heard this before, please listen to me: If you can make changes to avoid developing diabetes, you should put forth your best effort to do this. Diabetes is a beat that just does not stop, and it can become overwhelming and very tiring. **Hopefully, after reading further, you will realize why you are having so much trouble and the process may become a lot easier.**

If You Are Having a Hard Time with Diabetes Control

People who do not have diabetes do not understand everything that is involved. Some people think it is easy and that you just have to stay away from sugar. What many people do not realize is that it's not that simple; many factors help regulate blood sugar. It is complex, so do not feel bad if you are having trouble understanding it all. Being diagnosed with diabetes is traumatizing. You are being told that you have a disease that will never go away. You will have to take pills, wear a pump, or give yourself insulin shots daily for the rest of your life. Monitoring your blood sugar numbers throughout the day with a blood sugar monitor and pricking your finger to get the result will also become a daily chore. This means you will have to carry your supplies with you wherever you go and you have to go for quarterly doctor checkups. There will also be no choice but to eat differently, and you must be careful when participating in sports and strenuous activities.

This should not be used as an excuse to *avoid* exercise. You don't want your levels to drop too low from being active, *but* you most definitely do not want to be inactive. At this point, you might be wondering who can learn all of that when they are baffled by the news of becoming insulin-dependent. You may be feeling overwhelmed, but it is crucial to realize that it is possible to learn, understand, and master all of this.

Think about all the professional athletes in sports that have diabetes like Kendall Simmons, the former corner for the Pittsburgh Steelers, Jonathan Hayes is an American football coach, former tight end and author, Sam Fuld outfielder for the Tampa Bay Rays, Jay Cutler, quarterback for the Chicago Bears, Pamela Fernandes an Olympic Gold Medal Cyclist, Will Cross a Mountain Climber, and many more. For them, it takes plenty of "paying attention" to their body, learning by recording their numbers and being consistent with their care, but it is possible. Just like them, you need to put in some time to learn about food and lifestyle. This book is a great start for you!

There Is Not Enough Diabetes Education Available

The degree of education about food and nutrition that a person receives after being diagnosed with diabetes may not be enough initially. Every hospital is different, but if you feel that you did not receive enough education, then you need to make an effort to learn and contact your doctor. Take any food, nutrition, and/or diabetes education classes that they have to offer. My husband and I took classes, read tons of books, and researched information online for years. You may be offered classes after first being diagnosed and then you are on your own unless you request more. Your health is the most important part of your life, right? Often, education must be requested by your doctor to be covered under your insurance. If your diabetes doctor/hospital only has one educator and that person has not helped you, then you are out of luck unless you can pay for another educator, and it may not be covered by your insurance. All of this is another reason for you to read books, watch videos, and get online.

Keep an open mind when learning about diabetes and nutrition because there are many philosophies about control. Everyone is different and I found that if you learn as much as you can and keep your mind open, you can then apply the methods that help you best. Know that you can make decisions; tell your doctor what you think, and see if they will work with you. Diabetes medications keep changing with new improvements, different types of pumps and monitors, and the types of insulin available. Diet concepts are always changing. It can become a full-time job to educate yourself on these issues. Take your time and try not to overwhelm yourself, but do not quit.

Literature Cited in this Chapter

1. https://www.cbsnews.com/boston/pictures/awareness-month-famous-athletes-with-diabetes/11/
2. https://www.cnn.com/2017/05/05/health/diabetes-liebermann/index.html
3. https://www.healthline.com/diabetesmine/26-famous-people-with-type-1-diabetes#Athletes

Chapter 3

Observation – For Those with Diabetes AND Those Without Diabetes

The way that I was instructed to take care of my daughter's diabetes at 19 months old was a concept called the 360 Test, meaning full coverage throughout the day—basically, testing a lot. I was taught to check her blood sugar before each meal and snack and document the number and what she ate or was about to eat. I kept a steno notebook on the kitchen counter for this purpose (there are many Apps and online ways to keep track now). This may seem like an exhausting daily task, but if you want to understand what food does to your blood sugar, this is the way to learn. You may feel bad when you check your finger and the number is high; it may discourage you from wanting to check. When you check and the number is higher than you would like, write down the number and what you ate next to it. Next time, when you plan on eating that particular food again, you will remember the previous results and maybe incorporate some exercise after, or have water instead of a sugary drink with the meal. **This is where your education begins—by checking and remembering.**

You must learn what foods affect your blood sugar. Whether you are using an App, laptop, or a stenography notebook, you need to document the results. If every meal is too much for you to document, try one daily; and if that is too much, try a few times a week. Documentation is a necessity to be able to learn about how food affects your body. After a few months of documenting numbers and foods, you will probably be able to see patterns and you might even want to eliminate certain foods from your diet that skyrocket your blood sugar. Or, you may view them differently and only eat them as a "treat," once in a while, instead of often. In this book, I will make reference to the 360 test or this type of monitoring to let you know what I learned about food, which foods I've found to be hazardous, and, basically, my most valuable results from over a decade of documenting.

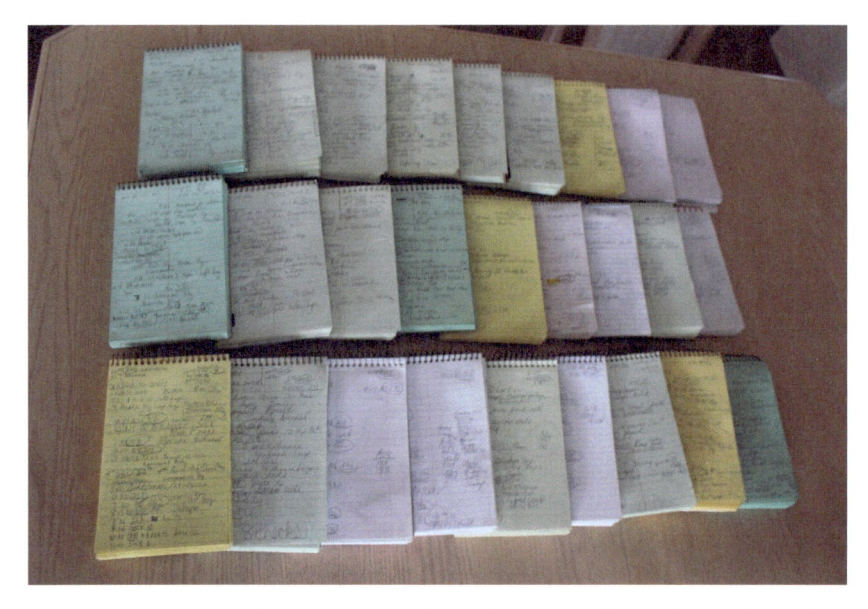

A person without diabetes may think this doesn't apply to them because they do not need to check their finger; however, consider this:

360 Test for A Person Without Diabetes: Embrace the Scale and Document

The scale can be used as a form of measurement, just as the 360 test uses numbers from blood sugar monitoring. Most recently, in our society, the scale has developed a bad reputation. The scale is not evil. Scale, by definition, is a balance or any various instrument or device for weighing. Scales are used daily in just about every industry. They hold great importance in our society. Some examples are the airline industry (to weigh baggage), the food industry (packaging), logistics (truck weight), weather (severity of storms and earthquakes), medical (amounts of medicine to be given and vitals of humans), education (to measure intelligence), utilities (how much we use), the list is endless. However, many humans refuse to use a scale, daily or weekly, to gauge their weight. It was a popular method in previous centuries but suddenly it is a forbidden practice for some. We hear comments like "Don't get on the scale daily, it's too depressing" and "Learn to embrace yourself and love the way you are, you don't need to weigh yourself."

Just as many industries in the U.S. rely on scales, I do too! I use the scale as a way to monitor and keep my weight in a 10-pound range. I wake up every day and at some point, I get on the scale before I eat. If I am on the low side of my range, I feel good and I know that if I do want dessert, I can afford to have it. If I am on the heavier side of my range, I know that there are a few things I must do and not do. In a way, I am keeping myself in-check like my daughter is.

Here are 10 of my personal tips when the scale is on the high end:

1. Substitute a carbohydrate meal for a salad (croutons or small pieces of bread are all right).

2. Skip desserts or have just a bite of something sweet (a piece of chocolate, a fun-size candy bar).

3. Replace a sugary drink with water.

4. Avoid any mega sugary drinks, such as coffee shop specialty coffees with added syrup.

5. Good things come to those who wait, and I promise myself to have whatever I want when I get back to the low range on the scale.

6. Depending on how high I am in my range, I may skip going out to eat, because restaurant meals often have higher salt, sugar, and fat and are of a larger portion.

7. If I do go out to eat, I will skip breaded and fried foods and go for a broiled or baked dish. I will also skip creamed soups and Alfredo, or any type of rich creamy dish.

8. If I feel the need to have a late-night snack, I will go for something very light, such as veggies and dip, instead of crackers or chips and dip.

9. Increase activity and or exercise.

10. I will choose a ONE-carbohydrate meal and, definitely, not combine two carbohydrates for a meal if I am higher in my range. *Vegetables are carbohydrates; however, most of them (except for starchy carbs such as potatoes) are low in carbs so they are often counted as "free" in the diet and diabetes world.*

Examples of one-carbohydrate meals:

- Pasta, chicken and vegetable
- Rice, meat, and vegetable
- Potatoes, meat and vegetable
- Burrito with meat and veggies (no potatoes or rice)

Taco and soup with no or few carbs, such as tortilla soup, wedding soup, or tomato soup.

Examples of two-carb meals that I avoid if I am higher on the scale:

- Breaded chicken or fish and French fries
- Hamburger and French fries
- Any sandwich and French fries
- Pasta, chicken/meat, and bread
- Rice, chicken/meat, and bread

Combining any two of these in any way: rice, potatoes, corn, wheat (bread, tacos, burritos, pizza, and or pasta) would be a two-carb meal.

I am also a huge fan of the "construction worker" breakfast (eggs, sausage or bacon, home fries or hash browns, and toast); if I am on the higher side of my range, I will choose to eat a less hearty breakfast, such as cereal and fruit or oatmeal and yogurt or eggs, and meat but no bread/toast.

During days when I am on the higher side of my range, I also make it a point to not lie around. I will try to get up and stay busy with cleaning, exercising, or going out for a walk. Especially before bed!

In conclusion, to learn about food and how it affects your body, you need some sort of measurement system to monitor yourself, and you need to pay attention and document results so that you remember and learn. If you are not willing to do this, your struggle with your weight and/or diabetes will be difficult. Whether you are using blood sugar numbers/averages or a scale to monitor yourself, you can be successful.

Chapter 4

Eliminate Unhealthy Self-Image Thinking

Before I explain the details of the four concepts that will help you obtain optimal results with your diet or diabetes management, I want to encourage and excite you for success with better health and weight physically, and also mentally. Your success will certainly have a positive impact on your mental state, specifically your self-esteem and self-image.

However, your current self-esteem and self-image may be a deterrent to your success. Some people who are overweight feel very good about themselves, focusing on their accomplishments and success in life while others struggle mentally and worry about what others may think of them.

Being bullied, whether as a child, teen or adult, can cause low self-esteem and self-image issues and mold how we perceive ourselves. Over time we can even come to expect negativity and may succumb to a label or become paranoid, frustrated, angry, or upset.

Awareness of difficult emotions is a big step toward making a successful life change. Negative thoughts can get in the way of success and accomplishing goals. When you are suffering, you may adopt a "why bother" attitude or be inclined to quit. It is important to recognize negative thoughts and dismantle them immediately.

This book will teach you how to change your diet and that takes time. During this time, people may try to bully you, judge you, or try to convince you to stop. The loud voice of self-doubt and insecurity can be persistent, discouraging, or even destructive to your efforts. We can all resonate with poisonous self-talk that invades different areas of our lives. Fear of being judged or rejected might make you shy away from people. You may stop doing things you enjoy or things that you want to accomplish. Some think this is just a problem in grade school and high school and do not realize that being teased and/or bullied about body size can continue into adulthood and create lifelong low self-esteem.

You may have heard the philosophy "accept who you are." However, if you know someone who is overweight, you may see that they have tried every diet out there (South Beach Diet, Weight Watchers, Mediterranean Diet, The Zone Diet, Atkins Diet, Paleo Diet, 21-Day Fix, and many more) with the hope of making a change. They may have also had a doctor warn them of the repercussions of extra weight and they may worry about their health. Their self-esteem and self-image may not be positive. So how can they accept and be happy with their body shape if it is affecting them on the inside? Someone in this position, who is trying to make a change in their diet to lose weight, may be vulnerable to negative comments and actions and could be easily convinced to abandon their efforts. Negative thoughts can hinder your success, so creating a positive self-image and self-esteem to accompany you in achieving your life goals, including weight loss, is immeasurable.

Fashion and Self-Esteem/Self-Image History

Looking at our history is vitally important to understand change and prepare for progress. It is a great way to prevent and/or correct mistakes. To understand the current self-esteem and self-image issues in the U.S., it is helpful to look at the history of fashion and the role it has played in self-perception.

I was at a family party where there was a beautiful black-and-white photo of a baseball park in Pittsburgh, PA called Forbes Field. When I asked my dad a question about the stadium, he answered and then added: "That's when people used to get dressed up to go to sporting events."

Actually, people used to dress up to go to church, work, parties, and funerals and on airplanes. In the previous century, each decade was defined by a certain style of clothing. In the early 1900s, for example, the high collar and very tight waistline dominated. By the 50s fashion returned to the tight waist on the long skirt and a short sweater. The mini-skirt and the bikini made their first appearance in the 1960s, taking fashion to a revealing level. But over time, something happened. The economy took off at a very fast pace, people were making money!

Everything was moving at an erratic pace. Women were entering fields that were previously dominated by men. How did this affect fashion? Tennis shoes entered the business world, for the first time, women were seen on the streets in business suits and tennis shoes. With the booming economy and the ability to spend, the trends became seasonal instead of yearly. Fashion was changing so quickly that it was not worth the investment for some.

Other interests such as computers, mobile phones, and other electronics became more important and more fun to invest in. And so, the "style" of the 90s became "loose" clothing that did not pack a punch for building self-esteem and self-image.

Technology has also allowed many people to work from home, some never changing from their pajamas to do a day's work. Loose clothing is user-friendly for food bingeing and weight gain.

Am I Really Overweight?

What is even more troubling is the confusion over what is overweight and what is fit. Sometimes "average" is considered normal. With the growth in numbers of obese people in the U.S. comes a development or perception of normalcy for obesity, leaving our youth confused as to why they are taunted for being overweight.

This perception has made the mirror become an invalid tool of measurement. To me, this is the scariest part of the current problem, especially when someone in the media and entertainment industry suffers abuse for flattering the fit and then becomes the target of negative remarks. What is seen in the entertainment and news industry can easily transfer to the school and workplace environment.

Heal Your Self-Esteem

The truth is that bullying has existed for centuries and isn't going away; in fact, social media has made it worse. It is much easier to say mean and insulting things to a person without facing them. As an overweight person, you may suffer abuse from co-workers, classmates, bullies, and even teachers and family members. If you had the chance to eliminate this, do you think it would help your self-esteem? The logical answer is yes. If you shed the extra weight, do you think that you would feel better mentally and physically? Do you think it would be easier to ignore bullies? Do you think that you may be able to participate in sports with more energy? The answer to these questions is <u>yes</u>.

Any amount of weight loss on the scale puts a smile on your face and makes you feel better. Being able to fit into clothes that you could not fit into a year ago makes you happy and more confident. Being fit is good for your self-image and your confidence. Being bullied is not good for you and not good for your self-esteem. Some basic steps to prevent your mental state from being damaged are:

- Ignore, block, and avoid negative people/negative encounters—walk away if you can because you aren't the problem, something else is bothering them.
- If you cannot get away, tell the negative person this behavior is serious and harmful.
- Stay calm—losing control will most likely not be helpful.
- Be confident and hold your head high—you are on a mission.
- Talk about how you feel with a counselor or someone positive.
- Eliminate negative people in your life and add positive people.
- Stand up for others that you see encountering negativity.
- Find role models who have gone through what you are going through.

In conclusion, knowing that weight loss will help your self-image and self-esteem and boost your confidence it is important to block out any negative energy from others or internally. If you have been brainwashed into thinking negative thoughts about yourself or if you anticipate them from others, it is time to wipe the slate clean. Stay focused and goal-driven. It will help you accomplish success. Set small goals to help you through this process.

Working hard through small goals can help you achieve large goals. You will find many small goals in this book that you can focus on. Instead of setting a goal of losing 50 pounds, think of packing a healthy lunch once a week or changing from a 32-ounce soda/sugar drink at lunch to a 12-ounce drink and stick with it.

Take small steps that you know you can easily accomplish and filter out the negative thoughts. Imagine a shield or reflective screen that deflects bullying or negative judgment.

Use this affirmation: "I am on a mission to make a positive change and I am going to succeed."

Refer back to this chapter every once in a while to remind yourself of your strength and desire. Imagine yourself as a character in a book or movie who is on a mission to be successful, and you have others counting on you to succeed. Your success will pave a path of encouragement for others.

Chapter 5

Four Key Concepts – ABCTs

In all of my years of taking care of my daughter, I've concluded that there are four basic concepts about proper diet and good diabetes control that produce positive results—no matter what form of insulin delivery you are using. These four basic concepts are also MY cardinal rules for staying FIT and SLIM.

Avoid unhealthy high-fat (saturated and trans-fat) **and high-sugar foods.** There is an old saying that I am sure you have heard, that goes something like: "Too much of anything is no good." It could not be truer when it comes to fat and sugar in food.

When my daughter was a toddler, she was growing and very active. She had low blood sugar many times. Here is some inside information: One of the ways that I used to get her sugar up was with orange juice; however, kids like a variety, so, sometimes I would use chocolate or strawberry syrup in milk to boost her. This was always a sure thing for getting her "up" from a low of around 35 to well over 100. I would put a tablespoon in six ounces of milk. This is something to consider when you are asking for those "extra pumps" at your favorite coffee shop. Most high-fructose syrups have about 25 grams of sugar in a mere 2 tablespoons, nearly as much as in some 12-ounce drinks. In the last century, black coffee was the most popular. In this century, dumping tons of fat and sugar in your coffee is the new trend. Add up the sugar and fat in three cups of black coffee versus three cups of current-day cappuccinos or lattes. Some people are getting their daily recommended amount of sugar and fat just in their morning coffee. An example of extreme unhealthy high-fat consumption used to take place at many kids' birthday parties when the kids were served pepperoni pizza, fried chicken nuggets, or French fries, and cookie cake or cake and ice cream.

This is when blood sugar goes up like a helium balloon and it is difficult to bring down.

Be active and avoid being sedentary, especially after meals. Sitting for long periods or going to sleep after meals will not help your blood sugar drop. I have witnessed this via the 360 Test and results. Blood sugar has a hard time dropping when you are dormant. Consistent activity is a huge help in controlling blood sugar. Now, more than ever, it is hard to get active due to our electronic obsessions. They are truly amusing so why not pretend you are at an amusement park where every ride ends? Set the alarm on your phone as a *ride-over* reminder and then get up and do something else. Make a list of 10 things that you could do or enjoy or feel better about if they were accomplished. Hang the list up where you play on your electronic device. When the alarm goes off, look at the list. This is your motivation.

Consistency in dieting. Yes, it can be boring, but it really works well to eat similar meals with foods that have similar amounts of fat and sugar daily. Splurging and eating foods with super high fat (saturated/unhealthy trans-fat) or sugar now and then can cause swings in blood sugar. Think about what your choices are at home. If you have a wide range of unhealthy high-fat and high-sugar foods available to pick from, then you are going to have a wide range of blood sugar numbers, or for for someone without diabetes, peaks and valleys in your energy level. Think of it in wardrobe terms. If you are trying to dress conservatively, but you have vibrant clothes, you may not meet your goal. Keep your food supply in your home conservative in fat and sugar and you will meet your diabetes or dietary goals. Consistency in your daily activity is also a good idea to keep blood sugar under control. **Note:** When high fat is mentioned in this book, I am mostly referring to unhealthy high fat.

Timing. You can't get around it. If you have diabetes, you probably have been told to eat breakfast, lunch, dinner, and possibly something before bed. You may need a very small snack in between some meals, depending on how insulin-sensitive you are. Going without breakfast or skipping a meal, only to overeat later, is not a good choice. It is dangerous as it puts you on a roller coaster of blood sugar highs and lows and this is visual if monitoring using the 360 test. For people who do not have diabetes or take insulin, you may experience feelings of hyperactivity and then extreme drowsiness. Most machines, electronics, or anything man-made operate smoothly when consistency is incorporated. For example, a swimming pool is easy to keep clean until you forget to add chlorine. And you can't add too much either. Or think about when vehicles need gasoline. You can't drive on an empty tank or fill up when the tank is full. A pattern and consistency in behavior are going to help you with dieting as well as diabetes. Do not underestimate the appreciation that your body will have if you learn to eat breakfast, lunch, and dinner consistently at a similar time every day. I learned this through the 360 test, and I guarantee it will be helpful.

Wait a Minute

You are not "good to go" with these four concepts. That would be nice, but you must continue reading first!

CHAPTER 6

Roadblocks to the Four Key Concepts- ABCTs

The four concepts seem kind of easy to follow when you look at them on paper, but **you may run into some obstacles.** These obstacles can make your fight to maintain good blood sugar harder—and they also happen to be the same obstacles responsible for the current obesity and diabetes epidemic in America. Some people want to blame the obesity problem on one factor alone, such as fast food or soda. **The truth is that there is a multitude of reasons, and these obstacles can be pretty tough.** How tough? Tough enough to produce these results: According to the United States (U.S.) Centers for Disease Control and Prevention, more than one-third of U.S. adults (42.4%) are obese, and approximately 19% (or 12.5 million) children and adolescents aged 2–19 years were obese as of 2017–2018.[1] From the 1960s to the 1980s, the number of overweight or obese teens remained steady at about only 5%. I said a mere FIVE PERCENT. **However, that number has tripled since the 1980s,**[1] **which means that something has changed.** This is a troubling statistic. Not only do overweight teens suffer from social disapproval and reduced ability to participate in physical activities, but they are also at an elevated risk for serious health problems like cancer, heart disease, high blood pressure, and diabetes.

However, "Obesity-related conditions include heart disease, stroke, type 2 diabetes and certain types of cancer are among the leading causes of PREVENTABLE (emphasis added by the author), premature death."[1] **They are preventable because losing weight can be very helpful.**[2,3]

I was once purchasing an item at the mall from a young female cashier. She said to me, "You are tiny, like my mom." Then she said, "My dad is thin too, and I don't know where my genes came from." There are quite a few factors that could be responsible for her different frame; however, there have been many dietary changes over the last few decades that could also be the reason. I used this encounter as inspiration to write this book.

OK, What Changed?

What has happened to cause this obesity increase? Gradual change can go unnoticed for years and then, all of a sudden, it's noticeable but it is difficult to turn back. It is like a factory dumping its waste into a river thinking that no one will know. However, 20 other factories along that same river are also quietly dumping their waste into it. Soon it is visibly polluted but it's too late to do anything about it.

There are a variety of contributing factors that have created the current obesity problem in the United States. **One single factor alone cannot be blamed.** Some of these factors include fast food intake, over-sized proportions, eating out more frequently, increase of sugar and fat content in food, availability of snacks everywhere via vending machines and convenience stores, eating more frequently, an electronic boom that leads to a sedentary lifestyle, hours of homework preventing after school activity, not packing a lunch for school, quality of food in schools, treats in schools and during after-school activities, lack of walking, lack of gym class in schools, and a much busier schedule for kids and parents that makes it difficult for parents to be home to cook quality meals. Some of these factors were non-existent 50 years ago. This change has happened at a very slow pace.

If you were born after the 80s, you may not be aware that some above factors have drastically changed. Personally, as a child and into my teen years, I rarely ate fast food or oversized portions and was not often exposed to high-sugar or high-fat foods. There was also little availability of snacks everywhere via vending machines and convenience stores. I ate breakfast, lunch, and dinner, and I rarely snacked. We did not own electronics, I was very active, did not have a ton of homework. I packed a lunch for school or ate good-quality school lunches. I also did not experience an abundance of treats in school or during after-school activities. Back then, more kids walked to school and had gym twice a week until graduation. I helped my mom prepare home-cooked meals at least three days a week all through middle school and high school.

The following chapters offer a more in-depth look at how the culture of the United States has changed and how this has contributed to the current obesity and diabetes problem. I have dedicated a chapter to each factor, and it should be noted that they are not in any order of importance.

Literature Cited in this Chapter

1. Obesity. United States Centers for Disease Control and Prevention. https://www.cdc.gov/obesity/index.html

2. What a 5% Weight Loss Can Do For Your Health. WebMD. January 28, 2023. https://www.webmd.com/diet/ss/slideshow-five-percent-weight-loss

3. Prediabetes – Your Chance to Prevent Type 2 Diabetes. United States Centers for Disease Control and Prevention. December 18, 2023. https://www.cdc.gov/diabetes/prevention-type-2/prediabetes-prevent-type-2.html

CHAPTER 7

Fast Food – What You May Not Know

Forty years ago, there were fast-food restaurants, but not nearly as many as there are now. I remember going out to eat with my family twice a month, which was usually a Friday night and payday for my father. However, we did not go to a fast-food restaurant by today's standards; we went to a local restaurant where we sat down and were served by a waitress. We usually had fish sandwiches or fried shrimp with baked potatoes or French fries and/or a salad. Generally, the fish was fresh from the local fish market. It was not frozen with preservatives and a high amount of salt. My family did not consider fast food to be "going out to dinner."

My husband's story is similar. He grew up in New York City and went out to eat infrequently as a child. When his family did go out to eat, it was at local restaurants. He told me that for him and his family, the franchise chain restaurants were not considered a place to "go out to dinner."

What does this mean? Well, it seems that the idea of "going out to dinner" has changed. The concept of having a host seat you at a table that has a tablecloth, silverware, and cloth napkins and a server taking your order is no longer the only choice for a "dining out experience." The *order yourself, serve yourself, get your own condiments and seat yourself* concept is direct competition for dining out the old-fashioned way and it is a "get out of making food at home" ticket. Most of the time, it is less expensive than going to an actual restaurant and so it wins out against local restaurants. Many people do not have to wait until payday to have the "new dining experience" at the big fast-food chains. This new dining experience is actually the restaurants charging you to do their services for them. So, what am I saying? Now that our standards for an out-to-dinner experience are much lower and these fast-food restaurants are so inexpensive, we can "go out to dinner" much more. **If we could reset our standards and make a commitment to eat at healthier restaurants, which may be more expensive and may mean that we cannot go as frequently, we most likely would improve our health and lose weight over time.**

I asked my parents if they went out to dinner when they were children, and they both said they NEVER went out to dinner. They both remember going for ice cream, occasionally, and going to the candy store frequently for a piece of gum or a piece of hard candy. A piece, not a whole bag. Around age 11 or 12, in the late 1940s, they both had their first experience of going out to dinner. They could get pizza or footlong chili dogs, but it was not a daily or even weekly event. My mom said that the kids in her neighborhood enjoyed having fresh strawberries and fresh fruit right off the peach, apple, or plum trees when they were in season. Another treat was occasionally my mom's grandfather would make chocolate-covered cherries.

The Way It Is Now

There is much more fast food available than there was 30 years ago.[1-3] There are now over 25,000 fast-food chains in the U.S., an increase of more than 1,000% since 1970. THAT'S A LOT! It is pretty obvious that restaurant food has never been as readily accessible to people as it is now. (Please keep in mind that the statistics in this chapter will change over time and will not stay current but I want to provide a general idea about fast-food density.)

10 Largest Fast-Food Chains in the U.S. by Location *(these numbers change and positions alternate overtime)*

What are the 10 biggest fast-food chains in the United States?

1. Subway: 24,722 locations

2. McDonald's: 14,098 locations

3. Starbucks: 10,821 locations

4. Pizza Hut: 7,600 locations

5. Burger King: 7,231 locations

6. Dunkin' Donuts: 7,015 locations

7. Wendy's: 6,594 locations

8. Dairy Queen: 6,187 locations

9. Taco Bell: 5,670 locations

10. Domino's Pizza: 4,907 locations

How Many Locations Did These Restaurants Have 50 to 60 Years Ago?

Keep in mind that there are 48 states in the continental United States (Hawaii and Alaska excluded). Two of the restaurants in the following list did not have enough locations to have a restaurant in each state and Domino's Pizza did not emerge until 1983. If the restaurant had 1,000 locations, then they could have had roughly 20 restaurants per state. For example, how many McDonald's can you think of in your area? You can probably think of five just in your local area that you are familiar with. How many cities are there in your state? Imagine if there were only 20 McDonald's in your entire State. Would one be near you? If your state has five cities or towns, then there might have only been four McDonald's in your entire city or town. Can you imagine there only being four McDonald's in the Los Angeles or Miami areas? I have tried to imagine spreading out four McDonald's in my hometown of Pittsburgh, Pennsylvania. I would put one right in the downtown area and then I would want one in each suburb: north, south, east, and west. That requires five, so one of the suburbs would not have one. Most restaurants were probably not spread evenly among the cities/towns within a state. There were some cities and towns that just did not have a McDonald's. I just want to give you a visual idea of how sparse fast-food restaurants were back in the 1970s. Look at the figures below, compared to the figures above to see the drastic increase in fast-food restaurant locations.

Locations By Restaurant 40 Years Ago

1. Subway: 16 locations in 1974

2. McDonald's: 1,000 restaurants in 1968

3. Starbucks: 5 stores in 1982

4. Pizza Hut: 1,000 restaurants in 1971

5. Burger King: 275 locations in 1967

6. Dunkin' Donuts: just over 1,000 locations in 1979

7. Wendy's: 1,000 restaurants in 1978

8. Taco Bell: 868 restaurants in 1978 (which were sold to Pepsi Co, Inc.)

9. Kentucky Fried Chicken: just over 600 franchises in 1963

10. Domino's Pizza: 1,000 restaurants in 1983

Other Facts

In 1975, McDonald's opened its first drive-thru in Sierra Vista, Arizona. Chicken McNuggets were invented in 1979. If you were a teenager before 1975, you would never have experienced a drive-thru or Chicken McNuggets as a child or an early teen.

The information below shows a combination of how many fast-food restaurants are in certain cities. To put this information into perspective, Las Vegas is showing 683 fast-food restaurants in their city. This is more fast-food locations than Kentucky Fried Chicken had in all of the United States in 1963.

Fast Food Density

Top 10 Cities with the Highest Fast-Food Saturation

The Daily Beast looked at American cities with populations of over 200,000 and came up with a list of the 40 towns with the highest ratio of chain fast food restaurants to population.

Of the top 10 cities on the list, three—including list-topper Orlando—are in Florida. Las Vegas (#5) had the highest total number of fast-food eateries with 683 while Spokane (#9) had the fewest (158).

Also, in all but two of the cities in the top 10, Subway was the most prominent chain restaurant. Burger King was the most prominent chain in the two other cities.

Top 10 Fast-Food Restaurants According to The Daily Beast

1. Orlando, FL

Total fast-food restaurants: 463

Fast-food restaurants per 100,000 residents: 196.3

Most prominent chain: Subway

2. Louisville, KY

Total fast-food restaurants: 377

Fast-food restaurants per 100,000 residents: 147.1

Most prominent chain: Subway

3. Richmond, VA

Total fast-food restaurants: 274

Fast-food restaurants per 100,000 residents: 134.0

Most prominent chain: Subway

4. Miami, FL

Total fast-food restaurants: 535

Fast-food restaurants per 100,000 residents: 123.5

Most prominent chain: Burger King

5. Las Vegas, NV

Total fast-food restaurants: 683

Fast-food restaurants per 100,000 residents: 120.3

Most prominent chain: Subway

6. Tampa, FL

Fast-food restaurants per 100,000 residents: 100.0

Most prominent chain: Subway

7. Baton Rouge, LA

Total fast-food restaurants: 216

Fast-food restaurants per 100,000 residents: 95.8

Most prominent chain: Burger King

8. Cincinnati, OH

Total fast-food restaurants: 313

Fast-food restaurants per 100,000 residents: 94.0

Most prominent chain: Subway

9. Spokane, WA

Total fast-food restaurants: 158

Fast-food restaurants per 100,000 residents: 77.7

Most prominent chain: Subway

10. Birmingham, AL

Total fast-food restaurants: 168

Fast-food restaurants per 100,000 residents: 73.0

Most prominent chain: Subway

Why are Inexpensive, Fast-Food Restaurants Bad?

Fast-food restaurants have a lot of competition now, as you can see from the statistics above. Everywhere you go, there are multiple fast-food chains. They have to be competitive. Each restaurant wants its food to taste the best! How do you get food to taste sensational? **High fat** (saturated and trans-fats), **high sugar content, and high sodium** make fast food taste great! Sodium (salt) is a preservative as well as a flavor enhancer and is a necessity to prevent restaurant food from spoiling, especially when it is sitting out for hours waiting for customers to come and consume it. This is why when you go out to eat, several hours later you may be extremely thirsty. If you go out to eat frequently, you may not notice your extreme thirst because you may always be thirsty. I can tell you that I do not go out to eat too often, and this *extreme thirst* is something that I notice after I eat fast food/restaurant food. It also helps me judge a restaurant in terms of whether I will go back or not. Too much salt is bad for the body and if I feel like I'm in the Sahara Desert after a meal at a certain restaurant, I will most likely not return. When our family goes on vacation, I research restaurant menus before going so that we can have some healthy meals while we are away, and my daughter's blood sugar can remain steady.

What You Can Do

Here are a few thoughts that help me determine what kind of restaurants and fast-food locations I will visit:

1. Does the restaurant offer healthy options such as baked potatoes, vegetables, and/or rice as a side dish, or do they serve only breaded and fried food?

2. Can I get water or fresh brewed iced tea (unsweetened)?

3. Do they offer healthy salads?

4. Are their French fries coated? (Coated French fries contain a lot more sodium and are usually coated with wheat or corn starch.)

5. Does the restaurant offer grilled chicken or fish?

Post-Visit

After visiting a restaurant, I ask myself and make a mental note about:

1. Was I extremely thirsty after the visit?

2. What size drinks did they serve and was I able to order a small drink?

3. What were the portions like?

4. Did I pay too much for what I received?

5. Was the food excessively greasy?

6. How did the meal affect my daughter's blood sugar?

7. How was the overall quality of the food?

8. Did the restaurant punish me financially for substituting healthy choices for unhealthy choices? For example, substituting a bowl of chicken soup for French fries. Did I have to pay extra?

9. Was the scale reading high the next day for me (weight gain/water weight from high salt)?

I will not return to a restaurant if they score poorly on my post-visit evaluation.

Good Rules to Follow When Eating Out

Does the restaurant offer any healthy options? Avoid Unhealthy high fat! Even before I had a child with diabetes, I learned that I would not remain skinny if I ate foods that were labeled deep-fried, pan-fried, basted, batter-dipped, breaded, creamy, crispy, scalloped, Alfredo, or au gratin. These foods may contain very unhealthy fats, and/or high sodium. Go for the grilled, baked, broiled, steamed, or lightly breaded selections. Force yourself to eat healthily! You will be surprised that after a year or so, you will actually prefer healthy choices.

Limit your misbehavior! Balance, balance! Having a cheeseburger, French fries, and sweet tea could be rough on your blood sugar. Don't combine three big offenders! Change it up and have French fries and a salad with grilled chicken and an unsweetened tea with a little sugar in it. Or, instead of ordering French fries, fried chicken nuggets, and a soda, order fried chicken nuggets, plain salad, and unsweetened tea.

When eating out, order water or unsweetened iced tea. Okay, I cannot stress this enough. If you are going out to dinner, you will most likely be consuming more calories than if you ate at home. You can reduce some of that calorie intake by merely ordering water or unsweetened iced tea with your meal. Even if you put one or two packets of regular sugar in that iced tea, it will most likely still have way less sugar in it than the typical *sweet* tea or soda that most restaurants serve. I know this for a fact because if I take my daughter out to eat, and she orders the "sweet" tea with her meal, she will have high blood sugar numbers two hours later. If she orders an unsweetened tea and puts one or two packs of sugar in it, she will have a better numbers two hours later. Drinks can be a huge source of hidden sugar and calories. One 32-ounce regular cola packs roughly 91 grams of sugar and about 425 calories, which can quickly use up a big portion of your daily sugar and calorie intake. Drink water, lemon water, or unsweetened tea. I also find some sports drinks to be blood sugar-friendly as well. A pack of sugar contains roughly 2–4 grams of sugar. If you eat at a fast-food restaurant twice a week and replace your 32-ounce soda **with an unsweetened iced tea with two packs of sugar, you will reduce your yearly intake of sugar by roughly 9,464 grams! Get your calories from the food that you eat, not what you drink.**

Dressing and condiments on the side. Ask the server to deliver your high-fat condiments—salad dressing, mayo, and/or sour cream—on the side, so that you can control how much you put on. In one tablespoon of mayonnaise or butter, there can be roughly 10 grams of fat! There are 14 grams of fat in one tablespoon of oil. Why do we feel inclined to use that whole packet of butter or mayonnaise? You do not have to use it all and you can really cut back on your fat intake if you do hold off just a little. **If you go to a fast-food restaurant twice a week and you use only half the mayonnaise packet (eliminating one tablespoon from**

your diet) then, in one year, you will have removed a possible 1,040 grams of fat from your diet. Small changes add up. A healthy salad can quickly turn unhealthy when smothered in high-fat dressing and fried toppings, so choose a salad with fresh veggies, grilled toppings, and less dressing.

Get used to special ordering. You CAN change the make-up of the COMBO MEAL! You can often feel rushed when choosing your meal at fast-food restaurants. The number system for the meals is to assist the restaurant, not you! They can sell more food faster if you use the number system. "I'll take a number 6," takes a lot less time than saying, "I do not want a combo meal, I'll take a grilled chicken sandwich with the mayonnaise on the side and a house salad, with ranch dressing on the side and an unsweetened tea with two packs of sugar." If you are unfamiliar with the restaurant, you may have to search the menu for healthy items or replacement items before you order. This could take a while; you should not feel rushed. Is your health worth a little more time and a little more money? Yes!

Portion control: be humble! Look at how much you have chosen to eat. Your body is your temple and the only one that you have until your time on earth is done. Don't abuse your temple. If you still feel hungry immediately after you have eaten, know that you WON'T be hungry in a half hour. It is so convenient to get back in line at the fast-food counter and get more food, but this is where you need CONTROL. It takes time for your body to register that you have eaten. Stop before you feel like you're going to burst! You can do it.

Drink size. "This IS our small size!" Have you heard that? They are showing you a 32 oz. cup and saying that it is their small size. At that point, I ask for a child's cup. If you take the 32 oz. cup, you will most likely drink it all because it is there; that is a lot of calories to take in.

Too Many Evils Together: The Fast-Food Competition

With so many fast-food restaurants plotted on the U.S. map, competition to get patrons to come in resorts to almost anything from crazy tempting desserts to "never before" food creations adorning websites and advertising material everywhere you look. Triple cheese-stuffed pizza crust, triple-decker burgers, various foods on top of burgers, such as French fries, boneless wings, and pierogies, deep-fried cheeseburger, Hellman's mayonnaise in hamburgers, fried chicken nuggets inside a grilled cheese, donut breakfast sandwiches, deep-fried Twinkies and

Oreos, deep-fried ice cream, bacon on ice cream, ice cream on chocolate chip pancakes, s'mores pancakes, yogurt with multiple candy toppings, and churro dog desserts (cinnamon churro sitting inside a chocolate-glazed donut, which is topped with frozen yogurt, caramel, and chocolate). These high-calorie bombs are deadly for those who desire to be fit and those struggling with diabetes. They are a definite no-no for someone with pre-diabetes.

A sick feeling may come over you when you eat these crazy foods, which is most likely your blood sugar spiking or your pancreas working overtime. The frequency of these combination foods is a sure ticket to obesity and other health problems. A good way to put in perspective just how bad these foods are and combat the desire for these insane food combinations is to learn what your total calorie intake for a day should be (roughly), then look at the calories in one of these temptations. Most of them will take up half of your day's caloric intake, if not more. Another way to see the big picture is to determine how often you eat these foods, take the calories, and times it by the frequency. Maybe you eat a crazy dessert once a week, take the total calories of that dessert and multiply it by 52. Now find a lower-calorie option and do the same. For example, the calories of a regular slice of pizza times 52 versus the calories of a slice of triple cheese-stuffed pizza crust pizza. How many calories did you save by eating a regular piece of pizza? Did it really taste all that different? Don't fall for the crazy combos that are designed as a marketing tool to get you to spend your money at a specific restaurant. There is no concern for your health, just a desire for your money.

Celebrations

Having a daughter with Type 1 diabetes has been a real eye-opener. When she was younger and required 8 to 10 blood sugar checks to ensure good management, I was able to see how different foods affected her blood sugar. She would normally get three shots of insulin a day—breakfast, lunch, and dinner. If we ate fast food, I could usually count on having to give her an extra shot because of the unhealthy high fat in the fast food. Sugar affects the blood sugar, but fat does as well. Both may require you to give yourself more insulin if you are insulin dependent. If you are not insulin-dependent, you can count on your pancreas working overtime. Another challenge for us was birthday parties or any celebration. The person coordinating the party is most likely not thinking of offering a healthy meal. Often, if it is held at a restaurant or entertainment facility, the choice of food is what the place offers for parties, so the coordinator may not really have much say. This is often a place or event where the evils are thrown together. Here is another thought to consider.

When you think about diabetes, you might just think that someone with diabetes cannot eat a lot of sugar, but high fat affects your blood sugar, too. At first, it does not affect the blood sugar, but six hours later, the high fat *holds* your blood sugar, especially if you aren't very active after eating. So, eating unhealthy high fat at 6 p.m. is not a good choice for my daughter because it is going to *hold* her blood sugar and keep it from dropping when she goes to bed. Combine that having sugar before bed and her number may be sky-high. So, the unhealthy high fat can cause problems six hours later, if you are eating or drinking a lot of sugar. Many times, fast food has excess salt in it so it's highly likely that you may be drinking something to quench your thirst. Hopefully, it is water, but, if it is sugar, remember that earlier fat could be holding your blood sugar and now the sugary drink is going to spike it more. If you are not taking insulin and think that this doesn't apply to you because you produce your own insulin, that is correct. Your blood sugar will not rise as dangerously, BUT your pancreas will work double-time to keep your blood sugar down. It is running a marathon and over time, it may burn out and that is when you may be diagnosed with Type 2 diabetes. Unhealthy high fat and sugar make your pancreas sweat! Give your pancreas a break: avoid unhealthy high fat and high sugar content. It is a mind-over-matter situation.

If you are trying to lose weight, maintain weight, or have diabetes, AVOID putting these evils (high sugar content and high fat) together!

Too Many Evils Together: Make A Better Choice

Choose ice cream, cake, and water over ice cream, cake, and soda or juice.

Choose a burger and milkshake over a burger, French fries, and a milkshake.

Choose pasta, salad, and unsweetened iced tea over pasta, bread, and a high-sugar drink

Choose pizza, ice cream, and water over pizza, ice cream, and soda

More You Can Do

1. Educate yourself and your family about the dangers of eating foods that contain unhealthy high fat, high sugar content, and high salt content by looking at the labels and comparing them to healthier foods. Take your child to the grocery store and read the labels of products.

2. Resist the temptation. You can do it!

3. Customize your order to how you want it, not how the restaurant wants you to have it.

4. If you have small children, **purchase only one drink and ask for a second cup,** so that you can split the drink in half. I have been handed a 16 oz. drink for each kid and I say, "I asked for a small." "This is a small" is always the answer. I say, "You have to be kidding me?" and I look down at my tiny kids. After this had happened a few times, I started asking to see the small cup before I would order. I have been told, "We're not allowed to give a second cup." I started carrying cups in my car. You know if you give a kid that much soda, they might just drink it. Avoid it if you can.

5. Dilute those drinks. This is hard when you go out to eat, but at home, it is a common practice for me. Adding a half cup of water to a sweet tea usually does not change the taste that much. Insulin-dependent people and people with a diabetes diagnosis should be careful with diluting drinks due to carb and sugar counting.

Literature Cited in this Chapter

1. Fast Food. Food Empowerment Project. 2024. https://foodispower.org/access-health/fast-food/

2. The Fascinating History of McDonald's. The #Fact Site. December 1, 2023. https://www.thefactsite.com/mcdonalds-history/

3. The Number of McDonald's Locations in the United States, North America, and the World in 2022. USA Today. July 30, 2022. https://www.usatoday.com/story/money/business/2022/07/30/how-many-mcdonalds-us-world/10123086002/

Chapter 8

Shocking: Portion Increase

The Way it Used to Be and the Way it is Now

Both food and liquid portions used to be a lot smaller. What I find the most disturbing about portion sizes is that if you were born after the 90s, you may not realize that food portions have become much larger—often twice the size that they used to be. This is true for beverages as well. Super-sized meals did not start until the 80s. Most teenagers and young adults do not realize that these giant portions greatly exceed the United States Department of Agriculture standards for a single serving. Can young people really be held accountable for their obesity? They have been misled and unless they have had guidance from an older person or someone educated in nutrition that has paid attention to the change, then they have no idea why it is so hard for them to maintain an appropriate weight. Large quantities of cheap food have distorted our perceptions of what a typical meal is supposed to look like, and this has contributed to obesity in the United States. The change happened slowly and since restaurants have adjusted their dishes to accommodate (larger plates and cups), the change is not very apparent. Everything has increased in size: bakers use larger muf-

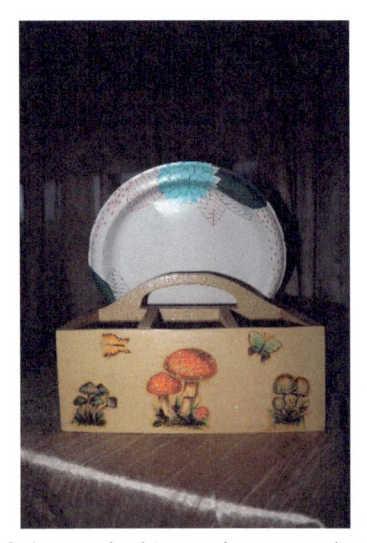

My father made this wooden paper plate holder for when my parents had family picnics. Many of today's paper plates are too large to sink into the holder properly.

fin tins and pie pans, pizzerias use larger pans, and the portion sizes in some cookbooks are larger.

Over-sized Portions When Eating Out

Our stomachs are about the size of an adult fist but can stretch to hold up to 4 liters. One liter is slightly less than 34 oz. If you drink a 32 oz (one liter) beverage and have a cheeseburger and fries, YOU ARE STRETCHING IT TO THE LIMIT! When the fast-food employee holds up that huge cup, LOOK AT YOUR FIST—that is your stomach; have some mercy.

A Look at Portion Sizes Then and Now *(The information in this section is subject to change over time. These examples are to provide a general idea about portion change.)*

Food/Beverage Portion Sizes in the 1950s vs Portion Sizes in 2014

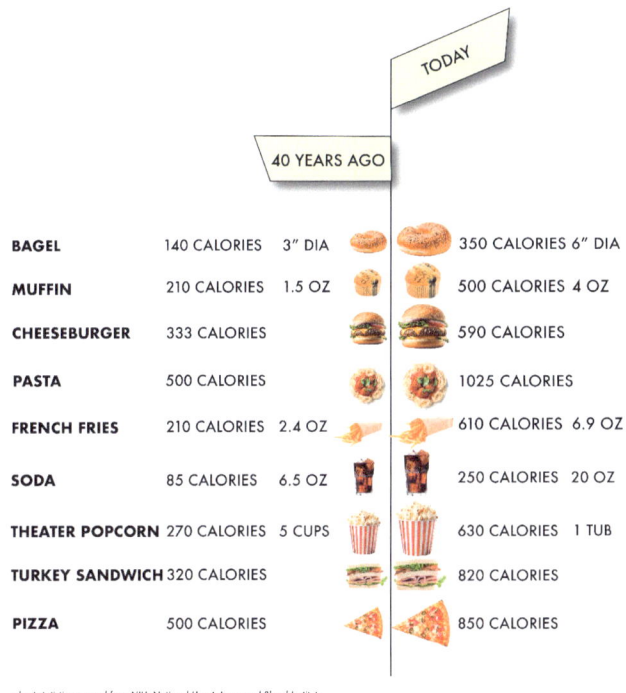

	40 YEARS AGO		TODAY
BAGEL	140 CALORIES 3" DIA		350 CALORIES 6" DIA
MUFFIN	210 CALORIES 1.5 OZ		500 CALORIES 4 OZ
CHEESEBURGER	333 CALORIES		590 CALORIES
PASTA	500 CALORIES		1025 CALORIES
FRENCH FRIES	210 CALORIES 2.4 OZ		610 CALORIES 6.9 OZ
SODA	85 CALORIES 6.5 OZ		250 CALORIES 20 OZ
THEATER POPCORN	270 CALORIES 5 CUPS		630 CALORIES 1 TUB
TURKEY SANDWICH	320 CALORIES		820 CALORIES
PIZZA	500 CALORIES		850 CALORIES

chart statistics sourced from NIH, National Heart, Lung, and Blood Institute

What You Can Do to Decrease Food Size and Intake

If you desire to lose weight or maintain a proper weight, you MUST recognize that portion sizes have increased, over time, to unhealthy levels and that you must eat smaller, more sensible portions. First of all, make sure that you have properly sized dishes and cups in your home. Today's plate size has increased to 12 inches in diameter, which is about 2 inches larger than it was in the 1980s. I recommend a 10-inch dinner plate, a 6-inch cereal and salad bowl, and an 8 oz. drinking glass to help control your portions. Get new dinnerware if you are currently using extra-large dishes!

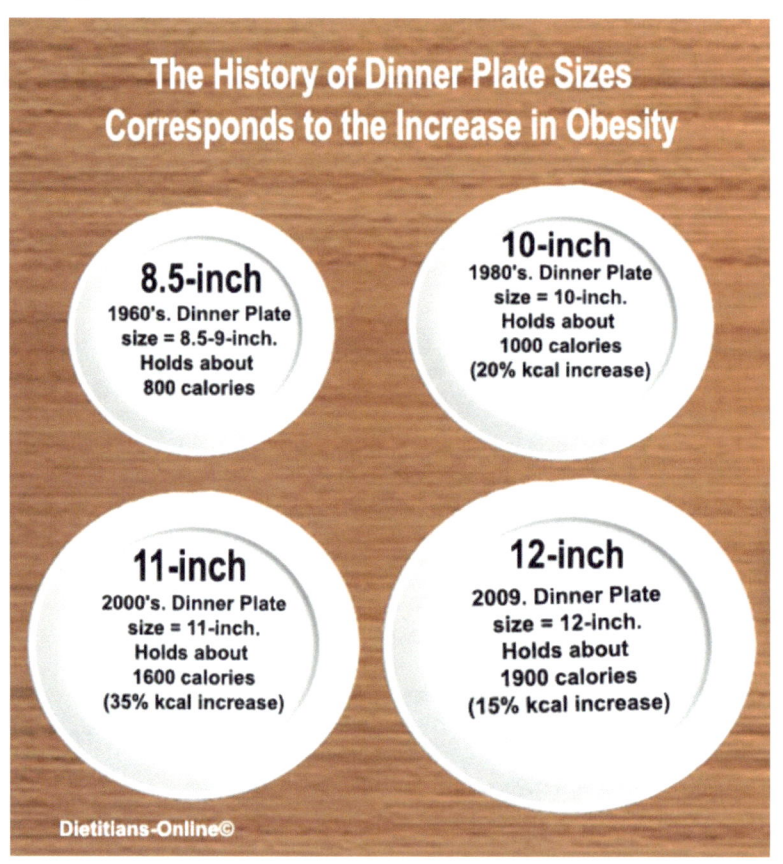

The History of Dinner Plate Sizes Corresponds to the Increase in Obesity

- **8.5-inch** — 1960's. Dinner Plate size = 8.5-9-inch. Holds about 800 calories
- **10-inch** — 1980's. Dinner Plate size = 10-inch. Holds about 1000 calories (20% kcal increase)
- **11-inch** — 2000's. Dinner Plate size = 11-inch. Holds about 1600 calories (35% kcal increase)
- **12-inch** — 2009. Dinner Plate size = 12-inch. Holds about 1900 calories (15% kcal increase)

Dietitians-Online©

Sandra Frank, Ed.D., RDN, FAND

Here are some more helpful tips that I use:

1. The Eat-Half Rule. Save half of your meal for the next day. This is very easy with a lot of foods: half a hoagie/sub/sandwich, half a bagel, half a quesadilla. Other foods are harder to divide: half of the pasta or rice dish.

2. Ask yourself when ordering, "Do I really need that much food?" Look at your fist as a reminder of the size of a normal stomach. In the last century, it was popular to get a "slice" (of pizza) and a drink. In this century, you CAN'T purchase just a slice of pizza at the majority of pizza shops; instead, you are forced to purchase at least a personal size or small pizza, which is probably three or four slices. It costs more and is way more than you need to eat in one sitting. If you can't find a pizza shop that will sell you just a slice, then get it in your head that you are going to eat only one or two slices of that small pizza, and then take the rest home or share it with someone else.

3. I do pay extra to avoid a combo meal at fast-food restaurants. Just ordering a sandwich and a drink can be more expensive than ordering a meal, but I do it. If I receive the French fries, I will most likely eat some of them, so I pay extra to not have them in my presence.

4. I ask for a small size cup when ordering fast food. If I am served a large cup full of iced tea (16 oz or more) or soda, I may keep sipping it; so, I ask for a small drink size. If a small isn't small enough, ask for the child's size.

5. Do not eat snacks from a bag! Put a couple of handfuls in a bowl and put the bag away.

6. Portion your snacks ahead of time after you buy them. Look at the serving size and put that amount into a Ziplock bag, so when you want to snack you'll eat a more appropriate amount instead of guesstimating.

7. Be cautious with salad dressing. We have all put too much dressing on a salad and then eat it anyway. You don't have to use the entire packet or container.

8. Some people "live to eat" and I can understand that. I love a delicious meal, but if I treated myself and feasted on my favorite foods all day long, I would not be fit or healthy. Sometimes, you have to "eat to live." Imagine if you were a person/pioneer in the 1700s. You really can survive on less food! You may currently eat three or four times what people ate in the 1700s. Cutting back a little should not be a problem.

9. Eat half and wait 20 minutes. It sounds hard, but it really isn't, if you are determined. If half is not enough, at first, then eat three-quarters of the meal and tell yourself you are going to save the rest for tomorrow. Close the lid or move the plate away from you and give it 20 minutes and I bet you will be able to wrap that portion up and put it in the fridge without eating it. It may not be enough for another dinner, however, it may make a nice breakfast or lunch along with a salad.

10. Do not let yourself get "wild-lion" hungry. Going over 5 hours without food likely means you are going to become very hungry and will want to gorge yourself. If you aren't an organized person, or if you are a person who doesn't give yourself enough time to eat breakfast before leaving the house, then you may be one of those people who get wild-lion hungry. You will most likely overeat when you get that first meal. Eating breakfast, lunch, and dinner will make a big difference in how hungry you feel. Get organized and make sure that your temple (your body) does not go long periods without food. That may mean getting up a little earlier to eat or packing a lunch for yourself!

Calorie Increase: The Way it Used to Be and the Way it is Now

When portion sizes increase, it's common sense that calories increase as well. If portions were smaller years ago, then calorie intake was lower.

What You Can Do

Understanding how many calories you SHOULD be consuming per day is just as important as understanding proper portion size. The chart below considers levels of activity, which is important to consider when estimating daily calorie intake:

Estimated Calorie Requirements

Calories for Gender Age (years) Sedentary Moderately Active

Guidelines are an important tool for all aspects of life and weight watching is no different. A suggested Calorie Chart from Health.gov[1,2] provides an estimate of what your daily calorie intake should be.

Estimated Calorie Needs per Day, by Age, Sex, and Physical Activity Level

The total number of calories a person needs each day varies depending on several factors, including the person's age, sex, height, weight, and level of physical activity. In addition, a need to lose, maintain, or gain weight and other factors affect how many calories should be consumed. Estimated amounts of calories needed to maintain calorie balance for various age and sex groups at three different levels of physical activity are provided. These estimates are based on the Estimated Energy Requirements (EER) equations, using reference heights (average) and reference weights (healthy) for each age-sex group. For children and adolescents, reference height and weight vary. For adults, the reference man is 5 feet 10 inches tall and weighs 154 pounds. The reference woman is 5 feet 4 inches tall and weighs 126 pounds.

Estimates range from 1,600 to 2,400 calories per day for adult women and 2,000 to 3,000 calories per day for adult men. Within each age and sex category, the low end of the range is for sedentary individuals; the high end of the range is for active individuals. Due to reductions in basal metabolic rate that occur with aging, calorie needs generally decrease for adults as they age. Estimated needs for young children range from 1,000 to 2,000 calories per day, and the range for older children and adolescents varies substantially from 1,400 to 3,200 calories per day, with boys generally having higher calorie needs than girls.

These are only estimates, and approximations of individual calorie needs can be aided with online tools such as those available at www.supertracker.usda.gov.[3]

MALES				FEMALES[d]			
AGE	Sedentary[a]	Moderately active[b]	Active[c]	AGE	Sedentary[a]	Moderately active[b]	Active[c]
2	1,000	1,000	1,000	2	1,000	1,000	1,000
3	1,000	1,400	1,400	3	1,000	1,200	1,400
4	1,200	1,400	1,600	4	1,200	1,400	1,400
5	1,200	1,400	1,600	5	1,200	1,400	1,600
6	1,400	1,600	1,800	6	1,200	1,400	1,600
7	1,400	1,600	1,800	7	1,200	1,600	1,800
8	1,400	1,600	2,000	8	1,400	1,600	1,800
9	1,600	1,800	2,000	9	1,400	1,600	1,800
10	1,600	1,800	2,200	10	1,400	1,800	2,000
11	1,800	2,000	2,200	11	1,600	1,800	2,000
12	1,800	2,200	2,400	12	1,600	2,000	2,200
13	2,000	2,200	2,600	13	1,600	2,000	2,200
14	2,000	2,400	2,800	14	1,800	2,000	2,400
15	2,200	2,600	3,000	15	1,800	2,000	2,400
16	2,400	2,800	3,200	16	1,800	2,000	2,400
17	2,400	2,800	3,200	17	1,800	2,000	2,400
18	2,400	2,800	3,200	18	1,800	2,000	2,400
19-20	2,600	2,800	3,000	19-20	2,000	2,200	2,400
21-25	2,400	2,800	3,000	21-25	2,000	2,200	2,400

AGE	Sedentary	Moderately active	Active	AGE	Sedentary	Moderately active	Active
26-30	2,400	2,600	3,000	26-30	1,800	2,000	2,400
31-35	2,400	2,600	3,000	31-35	1,800	2,000	2,200
36-40	2,400	2,600	2,800	36-40	1,800	2,000	2,200
41-45	2,200	2,600	2,800	41-45	1,800	2,000	2,200
46-50	2,200	2,400	2,800	46-50	1,800	2,000	2,200
51-55	2,200	2,400	2,800	51-55	1,600	1,800	2,200
56-60	2,200	2,400	2,600	56-60	1,600	1,800	2,200
61-65	2,000	2,400	2,600	61-65	1,600	1,800	2,000
66-70	2,000	2,200	2,600	66-70	1,600	1,800	2,000
71-75	2,000	2,200	2,600	71-75	1,600	1,800	2,000
76 and up	2,000	2,200	2,400	76 and up	1,600	1,800	2,000

Sedentary means a lifestyle that includes only the light physical activity associated with typical day-to-day life.

Moderately active means a lifestyle that includes physical activity equivalent to walking about 1.5 to 3 miles per day at 3 to 4 miles per hour, in addition to the light physical activity associated with typical day-to-day life.

Active means a lifestyle that includes physical activity equivalent to walking more than 3 miles per day at 3 to 4 miles per hour, in addition to the light physical activity associated with typical day-to-day life.[3]

A key to losing weight and/or staying fit and controlling diabetes is understanding how many calories you should be eating per day. Also, realize that modern-day food services may be serving you too-large portions, which can make counting calories and properly feeding your body more difficult. Adjusting these portions can be easy once you get used to remembering what you must do and doing it daily: portion awareness and proper calorie control.

Over-sized Drinks: The Way it Used to Be and the Way it is Now

I believe that oversized drinks are a large contributing factor to obesity, and I wanted to specifically dedicate a section to this issue. As mentioned earlier, drinks—as well as food—have increased dramatically in size over the past four decades. Drinks were never as abundant and as large as they are now. Drinks are loaded with more sugar and high-fructose corn syrup than ever before. The 8 oz juice glass has become extinct and replaced by the 16 to 32 oz fast-food paper cups. There are currently soda drinks available in 64 oz size! You just can't get an 8 oz cup today, which is all you need with a meal. You can ask for a child's size cup and it will most likely be 12 ounces. When I ask for a child's cup, I won't be tempted to drink 16 or more ounces. Control is the key, and you can do it too. You must realize that when SIZE increases, so do CARBOHYDRATES, CALORIES, and SUGAR! Drinks have almost become "adult pacifiers," with so many people just constantly sipping a huge drink that is loaded with calories and sugar. Remember how big your stomach is—around the size of your fist—so have mercy on your stomach, kidneys, and bladder, which must process all the liquid you drink.

What You Can Do

Here is a helpful list of tricks, considering some of the information that you have read so far, to help you meet your goals.

1. Remember how big your stomach is. Visualize that you are packing a suitcase when you receive your meal. A tennis ball is about the size of one cup, and this is about the right portion of milk, juice, canned fruit, or raw vegetables that a person should eat. The size and thickness of a person's palm is about the correct portion of meat, fish, a burger, chicken breast, pork chop, turkey, ham, or any other kind of meat, poultry, or fish that a person should eat. The tip of the thumb shows a portion of butter or margarine that should be used. Keep these sizes in mind and try to imagine how all the food will fit in your stomach. Next, look at your drink, which must fit too! Is there room for 64 oz of liquid?

2. Variety is the spice of life. When you pack your suitcase for a vacation, you most likely pack a variety of items, right? Same with your stomach. You may think that a piece of meat that is the size of the palm of your hand is not nearly enough to satisfy your appetite, but remember, a plate should be divided into three equal sections. One-third of the plate should be filled with a non-starchy vegetable, one-third should be filled with starches, grains, or pasta and one-third should contain a protein: meat, fish, poultry, eggs, dairy, or tofu. You wouldn't pack a suitcase for vacation with just blue jeans, right? You want a variety of clothing. Don't eat just a huge bowl of pasta or a huge steak. Make sure you get all your suggested nutrients. **Nutrition should trump huge nutritionally void drinks.** Pack the important stuff. Ask yourself if you would prefer your daily calories from a nutritionally void drink or some nutritional food.

3. Gradually decrease your drink size. Switching suddenly to the proper portion sizes may be a difficult task but cutting back slowly just a little at a time is probably more reasonable. Set goals for yourself, such as only one purchased drink a day and it must be 16 oz or less. You could switch from 64 ounces to 32, then 20, then 16, and finally 12. Gradual change is good.

4. Bring your own drink in the car, either water or something with less sugar than soda. I do this often and it is also a way to "refuse the combo." If you have a drink already then all you need to do is refuse to order the combo and ask for just a sandwich. This will save you money as well. If you get to the drive-thru and you don't have your own drink, then you will most likely need the combo. If you have your own drink, it is going to be easier to "refuse the combo" and just get a sandwich. Eliminating the French fries may be hard, but it is a big step to gaining control. Fighting the convenience of a combo meal is tough.

5. Get to know the calories, sugar, salt, fat, and natural or artificial ingredients in your favorite drinks. Sometimes it is easier to avoid something if you know exactly WHY it is bad for you. Look up the nutritional information for your favorite drink or combo meal! Yikes!

6. DON'T FINISH IT! It's that simple. You do not have to finish everything you eat. We have a strong desire to finish what we are eating. Stopping and wrapping it for tomorrow or throwing it away takes willpower.

7. Morning sweets. One trick that I've always practiced and that I recently found out my very fit neighbor also practices, is to save it for the morning. Often at evening parties, I will take a piece of cake or a cookie and save it for the morning. Tell co-workers who are pushing for you to join in on afternoon desserts that you would love to try it, but you are going to take it for the next morning when you wake up. You have a better chance of burning all the calories from a treat if you eat it in the morning or when you first start your day. Eating high fat or sugar in the afternoon, evening, or shortly before going to bed does not give your metabolism time to burn it off. While this may not be a concept that is taught in nutrition classes, it seems to work for me and my neighbor. Let's face it, total avoidance is difficult, so if you are going to cheat, do it when you are going to be active for a while. Regarding diabetes, it also works better than eating high fat and high sugar late at night when your insulin feed may be at its lowest for safety precautions.

8. Think of sweets and treats as dessert! When there is extreme availability, an item is no longer considered "special." It is the supply-and-demand concept. The *Scholastic Pocket Dictionary* says that "dessert" is "A food, such as ice cream, fruit or cake, usually served at the end of a meal." It does not say it is food that we eat all day long or four times a day or as a replacement for a meal. It does not say that it is a tool to help our kids learn or behave correctly in school or that it is used to reward. Understanding what a "treat" is will help you with your control. Teach yourself that dessert is a ONCE-a-day event—if that. Seeing what current-day smoothies, slushies, and iced coffees do to blood sugar, I would suggest avoiding them altogether, but if you are in a habit and enjoy them, at least try to curb your intake. Make your favorite sugary drink a once-a-week treat and then a once-a-month treat.

9. Replace sides or dessert with fruit. I went to lunch once with a fitness fanatic. He ordered a turkey sandwich and an apple. I told him that I never would have thought to do that. American fast-food chains have us convinced that fries or chips go with sandwiches, so we eat a two-carbohydrate meal. He said, "If you don't eat desserts, you won't believe how sweet this apple will taste." **Fruit will suppress your sugar craving after a meal.** Fruit may not always be available, but it is easy to carry, especially apples and raisins. Fruit is lower in sugar than most desserts (and doesn't contain high-fructose corn syrup) and it's very low in fat.

10. Dilute. It is a good idea to avoid buying highly sugary drinks but, if you do, try diluting them with a little water. Pour a ¼ cup of water into your cup and then add the sugary drink. It will not change the taste that much and every little bit helps. For dieters, over a period of a week and then a month you will have drastically reduced your sugar intake**.** If you have diabetes be cautious with diluting if you are counting carbs.

11. Drink black coffee or use skim milk for cream. For all of you coffee-shop junkies, the creams, syrups, and sugars in your coffee are hard on blood sugar and are a lot of extra sneaky calories.

12. Carb Cautious. For the bread-and-butter junkies, have you ever gone to a restaurant with the great intention to eat a healthy meal, and then you eat so much bread and butter before the meal that it's not so healthy anymore? If you know that you cannot pass up the bread before the meal then skip the carbs (potatoes, rice, pasta) with the meal. Instead of getting chicken parmesan and pasta, get chicken parmesan and broccoli or a salad – because you already had a carb. Don't be afraid to tell your server that you do not want a carb with the meal. You can get two vegetables or a vegetable and a salad with your meat or ask your server to box the pasta, potato, or rice to go. This way you will reduce your carbohydrate intake. If dessert is your kryptonite, skip the carb in the meal in exchange for the dessert!

Literature Cited in this Chapter

1. Dietary Guidelines for Americans. United States Department of Health and Human Services. April 1, 2024. https://health.gov/our-work/nutrition-physical-activity/dietary-guidelines

2. 2015 – 2020 Dietary Guidelines. United States Department of Health and Human Services, Office of Disease Prevention and Health Promotion. https://health.gov/our-work/nutrition-physical-activity/dietary-guidelines/previous-dietary-guidelines/2015

3. Supertracker. United States Department of Agriculture. January 8, 2015. https://www.usda.gov/media/blog/archive/tag/supertracker.usda.gov

4. Food/Beverage Portion Sizes in the 1950s vs Portion Sizes in 2014

4. https://www.nhlbi.nih.gov/health/educational/wecan/portion/menuview.htm

5. https://www.freepik.com/

Chapter 9

Explosion of Food Processing and Packaged Food

Primary food processing is the transformation of raw foods, agricultural products, or animals into accessible food. Food processing includes all procedures that alter the food from its natural state. Minimally processed foods retain their original properties in nutrition, physical, sensory, and chemical properties (vitamins and nutrients) can be subjected to secondary processing. Examples of primary processing are milling wheat, the pasteurization of milk, and the sorting and refrigeration of meat. These foods may be minimally altered by removal of inedible or unwanted parts, drying, crushing, roasting, boiling, or freezing to make them suitable to store and safe to consume. Some examples of minimally processed foods would include fruit and vegetables, fresh meat and fish, dairy products and sauces, and raw unsalted nuts.

Secondary food processing changes food from its natural or raw state into more useful or edible forms. These foods are refined, purified, extracted, milled, dehydrated, or hydrogenated. Examples of secondary food products are processed: cheese and yogurt, flour, edible oils, canned fish or canned vegetables, fruits in syrup, and freshly made bread and cereal. These foods are essentially made by adding or combining salt, oil, sugar, or other substances. Most secondary processed foods have two or three ingredients and include packaging. Some secondary foods may contain chemicals to extend shelf life, protection from heat, and physical, chemical, and biological deterioration.

Tertiary food processing or ultra-processed foods are highly processed or ultra-processed. They are produced by combining primary food products and other secondary food products to create ready-to-eat food and drink products with a high sensory appeal (often using flashy packaging and names) like cakes, snacks, sweets, and heat-and-eat meals. They most likely have many added ingredients such as sugar, salt, fat, and artificial colors or preservatives. Ultra-processed foods are made mostly from substances extracted from foods, such as fats, starches, added sugars, and hydrogenated fats. They may also contain additives such as artificial colors and flavors or stabilizers. Like secondary food processing, these ultra-processed foods will contain chemicals to extend shelf life and protect them from heat, and physical, chemical, and biological deterioration. They are multi-ingredient foods that are no longer recognizable as their original source. More examples are bread, cookies, crisps, ready meals, pizza, chips, cereals, sweets, fizzy drinks, frozen meals, soft drinks, hot dogs and cold cuts, fast food, packaged cookies, and salty snacks. Ultra-processed foods are easily recognizable by their paragraph of ingredients!

They also are a large part of the typical Western Diet. Sixty percent of the American diet consists of foods from these categories.[1] Highly processed foods are designed to be addictive with high sugar, salt, and fat content. They taste good! Cookies, ice cream, pizza, and chips, for the majority, taste much better than grilled chicken, rice, steamed vegetables, and water.

Whenever possible, try to avoid or limit ultra-processed foods. Consider the examples in this table to help you quickly determine if food is minimally processed, processed, or ultra-processed.

Good examples of unprocessed, processed, and ultra-processed food (the NOVA system[2]) can be found in a recent article published in *The New York Times*.[3]

Nutritional Science -- What You May Not Know

Food Processing with Food Fortification is Extremely Helpful - **Improved Food Processing and Nutritional Science Played a Huge Role in the Elimination of Disease.**

Before researching to write this chapter, I was under the assumption that vaccines were what eliminated many of the diseases from previous centuries. These diseases were not around in the latter half of the 1900s. I was surprised to learn that achievements in public health, such as better food processing and nutritional science played a huge role in reducing cases and/or eliminating some diseases.

Read the statement below from *Achievements in Public Health, 1900-1999: Safer and Healthier Foods*[4] to see the history of secondary food processing and how it played a huge role in the reduction of disease in the 1900s.

Achievements in Public Health, 1900-1999: Safer and Healthier Foods

During the early 20th century, contaminated food, milk, and water caused many foodborne infections, including typhoid fever, tuberculosis, botulism, and scarlet fever. In 1906, Upton Sinclair described in his novel The Jungle the unwholesome working environment in the Chicago meat-packing industry and the unsanitary conditions under which food was produced.

I was surprised to learn that achievements in public health, such as **better food processing** and **nutritional science** played a huge role in reducing cases and/or eliminating some diseases. During the early 20th century, contaminated food, milk, and water caused many food-borne infections, including **typhoid fever, tuberculosis, botulism, and scarlet fever.** In 1906, the first consumer protection law was developed, the Pure Food and Drug Act, to regulate the quality of food and food processing to avoid the spread of food-borne diseases. Once the sources and characteristics of food-borne diseases were identified—long before vaccines or antibiotics—they could be controlled by hand washing, sanitation, refrigeration, pasteurization, and pesticide application. Healthier animal care, feeding, and processing also improved food supply safety. For example, in 1900, the incidence of typhoid fever (a bacterial disease spread through contaminated food and water or close contact) was approximately 100 per 100,000 (population); by 1920, it had decreased to 33.8, and by 1960 it was considered very rare.

It wasn't until the late 1800s that theories about **nutritional science** were taken seriously. It was discovered that **minerals and vitamins** were necessary to prevent diseases caused by dietary deficiencies. Recurring nutritional deficiency diseases, including **rickets, scurvy, beriberi, and pellagra** were thought to be infectious diseases. By 1900, biochemists and physiologists had identified protein, fat, and carbohydrates as the basic nutrients in food. By 1916, new data had led to the discovery that food contained vitamins, and the lack of vitamins could cause disease. These scientific discoveries and the resulting public health policies, such as **food fortification programs (the addition of nutrients to food),** led to substantial reductions in nutritional deficiency diseases during the first half of the century.

Food Fortification -- The Addition of Nutrients to Food

Also from *Achievements in Public Health*[4]:

The discovery of essential nutrients and their roles in disease prevention has been instrumental in nearly eliminating nutritional deficiency diseases such as **goiter, rickets, and pellagra** in the United States. During 1922–1927, with the implementation of a statewide prevention program, the goiter rate in Michigan fell from 38.6% to 9.0 %. In 1921, rickets was considered the most common nutritional disease of children, affecting approximately 75% of infants in New York City. In the 1940s, the fortification of milk with vitamin D was a critical step in rickets control.

Because of food restrictions and shortages during the First World War, scientific discoveries in nutrition were translated quickly into public health policy; in 1917, USDA issued the first dietary recommendations based on five food groups; in 1924, iodine was added to salt to prevent goiter. The 1921–1929 Maternal and Infancy Act enabled state health departments to employ nutritionists, and during the 1930s, the federal government developed food relief and food commodity distribution programs, including school feeding and nutrition education programs, and national food consumption surveys.

Pellagra is also a good example of the translation of scientific understanding to public health action to prevent nutritional deficiency. Pellagra is a dietary deficiency disease caused by insufficient niacin. Then considered infectious, it was known as the disease of the four Ds: diarrhea, dermatitis, dementia, and death. The first outbreak was reported in 1907. In 1909, more than 1,000 cases were estimated based on reports from 13 states. One year later, approximately 3,000 cases were suspected nationwide based on estimates from 30 states and the District of Columbia. By the end of 1911, pellagra had been reported in all but 9 states, and prevalence estimates had increased nearly nine-fold. During 1906–1940, approximately 3 million cases and approximately 100,000 deaths were attributed to pellagra. From 1914 until his death in 1929, Joseph Goldberger, a Public Health Service physician, conducted groundbreaking studies that demonstrated that pellagra was not infectious but was associated with poverty and poor diet. Despite compelling evidence, his hypothesis remained controversial and unconfirmed until 1937. The near elimination of pellagra by the end of the 1940s has been attributed to improved diet and health associated with economic recovery during the 1940s and to the **enrichment of flour with niacin.** Today, most physicians in the United States have never seen pellagra although outbreaks continue to occur, particularly among refugees and during emergencies in developing countries.

The growth of publicly funded nutrition programs was accelerated during the early 1940s because of reports that 25% of draftees showed evidence of past or present malnutrition; a frequent cause of rejection from military service was tooth decay or loss. In 1941, President Franklin D. Roosevelt convened the National Nutrition Conference for Defense, which led to the first recommended dietary allowances of nutrients and resulted in the issuance of War Order Number One, a program to **enrich wheat flour with vitamins and iron.** In 1998, the most recent food fortification program was initiated; **folic acid, a water-soluble vitamin,** was added to cereal and grain products to prevent neural tube defects.

While the first half of the century was devoted to preventing and controlling nutritional deficiency disease, the focus of the second half of the 1900s was to control chronic conditions, such as cardiovascular disease and obesity. An important challenge to nutritional health during the 21st century is obesity. In the United States, with an abundant, inexpensive food supply and a largely sedentary population, over-nutrition has become an important contributor to morbidity and mortality in adults and children.

What we consume is super important to our health! The food we consume supports our body's immune system with how well it performs to prevent you from getting diseases, viruses, colds, influenza, etc. There is truth to the saying, "You are what you eat."

In my opinion, from 1940 to 1980, real food was eaten. With primary and secondary food being fortified (but without as many preservatives and chemicals) and ultra-processed foods not on the market yet, our diet was very healthy. Many chemicals and additives in ultra-processed foods are not recognized by our bodies as nutrients. **A person who eats a lot of ultra-processed foods may actually have nutritional deficiencies that are similar to those developed by people who lived before food fortification existed.**[5]

End of 20th Century Explosion of Packaged and Processed Food

What caused the increase?

1. Taste and appearance became a marketing tool
2. Added nutrients/fortified with vitamins for health and energy also became a marketing tool
3. Longer shelf life
4. Convenience
5. Food supplier competition

In conjunction with the benefit of vitamins and minerals that processed and packaged food brought to the population, other positive attributes emerged such as convenience and longer shelf life. These latter two benefits not only made life easier for the general population, but they were also very beneficial to food suppliers. Longer shelf life meant less food would spoil on the shelf before being purchased, thus increasing profits. Also, the convenience of these products is a great selling feature. With consumers enjoying the **health benefits,** and food suppliers reaping the profits, the packaged and processed food business soared. By the mid-1900s, the market was becoming very **competitive.** The competition produced two more aspects: taste and appearance. The tastier the product was and the more appealing the appearance, the better the chances were of it being a big seller. By the end of the 20th century, many packaged and processed foods were loaded with preservatives (for longer shelf life) and taste-enhancing sugars, fats, and salts. Many chemicals were also added for appearance, preservation, and taste as well. This meant a lengthy amount of ingredients. Too much of anything is not good! **Most food additives now are not for nutritional purposes.**

What You Can Do

Stop the Addiction: 10 Quick Tips

Although this concept is not fully accepted by the medical community, some people believe that our brains get addicted to the effects of ultra-processed foods and that they elicit a response that is similar to that of a drug (i.e., rapid absorption, stimulation of pleasurable sensations, etc.) making it extremely hard to "diet." Based on this hypothesis, the importance of eliminating or reducing ultra-processed foods when trying to control your weight will be imperative to your success. Here is a quick set of instructions to help you to avoid the perils of the ultra-processed-food jungle.

1. Shop the perimeter of the grocery store. The perimeter of the grocery store usually stocks fresh and less processed foods. Along the perimeters, you will find more secondary processed foods. The middle of the store will have more ultra-processed foods like frozen food and snacks. Fill your shopping cart with foods from the perimeter of the store such as produce, dairy, nuts, freshly baked bread, meats, and seafood.

2. Buy fewer of the simple-carb products in the center of the grocery store because many of them are stripped of most of their nutrients. They contain empty calories and provide little nutritional benefit. Opt for complex carbs instead. Choose what you purchase from the center of the grocery store carefully, so you aren't buying too many ultra-processed foods.

3. Pass up any items with a paragraph-long list of ingredients!

4. Replace some ultra-processed foods with healthier alternatives. Trade super flavored tortilla chips for white tortilla chips (with fresh, healthy salsa to add nutrition), boxed mac and cheese for noodles with fresh Parmesan cheese, or instead of packaged apple pie, buy fresh fruit.

5. Cook more! Instead of frozen waffles make waffle and pancake mix from scratch, bread your own chicken fingers and freeze (there are videos online for breading chicken), make fresh popcorn at home in a pot on the stove (there are videos available online), and make cookies from scratch and freeze (they won't have all the preservatives and artificial ingredients in them). Instead of buying a frozen smoothie kit, make your own fresh fruit concoction or buy unsweetened frozen fruit chunks and add your own sugar if needed.

6. Don't fall for convenience. Shred cheese with a shredder; while this takes more time, you will avoid the anti-caking additives that are in store-bought shredded cheese bags.

7. Instead of opting for pre-made, purchase frozen meal ingredients separately. Make plain rice or buy frozen plain quinoa, frozen edamame or cauliflower, and frozen broccoli, and add your own sauce, cheese, meat, and flavorings, so you know all the ingredients going into your dish and you avoid the extra sugar, fat, and preservatives that are in frozen meals.

8. Check serving size because some frozen dinners are considered more than one serving which means if you look at the calories and nutrition facts on the packet, you will be eating double or triple that amount if you are eating the entire thing.

9. Spot red flags: high numbers for fat, sugar, and sodium on a package label aren't good so choose products with lower saturated fat, added sugars, and salt. I try to keep the amount of fat in the single digits for "each meal". It can be tricky because the package may say 6 g of fat but it may be for 2 tablespoons—like cream cheese. It is very easy to use more than 2 tablespoons of cream cheese. So watch the amount listed but also look at the serving size and try to limit fat to under 10 grams per meal.

10. Quality: choose a product with fiber, vitamins, and minerals. Avoid frozen products that have no protein or fiber. Protein and fiber keep you full.

Choosing Quality Processed Foods

Foods that are processed, packaged, and nutritional.

1. Healthy yogurt (not a lot of added sugar)
2. Canned beans (can be rinsed to reduce sodium)
3. Jarred spaghetti sauce (choose ones low in sugar and salt)
4. Oatmeal
5. Canned salmon
6. Peanut butter
7. Frozen vegetables
8. Granola bars (look for ones with less than 5 grams of sugar)

9. Dried fruit (look for ones with just fruit listed as the ingredient)
10. Fortified high-quality milk
11. Hummus
12. Cottage cheese

Eliminating some of the unhealthy processed foods from your diet can go a long way to helping you lose unwanted weight and giving you a healthier lifestyle altogether. Here is a short list of some unhealthy processed foods to avoid[6]:

- Sugary beverages such as sweetened coffee and tea, energy drinks, and soft drinks
- Deli meats, hot dogs and sausages
- Frozen pizza and frozen meals
- Packaged snacks such as chips, cookies, crackers and baked goods
- Most breakfast cereals
- Canned or instant soups
- Boxed instant pasta products
- Sweetened yogurt
- Bouillion cubes or paste

Eliminating highly-processed and ultra-processed foods completely is probably impossible; however, reducing your intake of these products daily can be very helpful to improve your diet. Realize that not every day can be a day of convenience and that some days we need to have a good home-cooked meal or pack a healthy lunch. Realizing that making a lifestyle change to incorporate the time and effort of preparing, and packing meals is a must, to improve our health and diet.

Literature Cited in this Chapter

1. Martinez-Steele E, Khandpur N, Batis C. *et al.* Best practices for applying the Nova food classification system. *Nature Food*. 2023; 4:445–448. doi:10.1038/s43016-023-00779-w

2. Callahan, A. How bad are ultraprocessed foods really? The New York Times. May 6, 2024, https://www.nytimes.com/2024/05/06/well/eat/ultraprocessed-foods-harmful-health.html

3. Achievements in Public Health, 1900-1999: Safer and Healthier Foods. United States Centers for Disease Control and Prevention Morbidity and Mortality Weekly Report. October 15, 1999. https://www.cdc.gov/mmwr/preview/mmwrhtml/mm4840a1.htm

4. Martini D, Godos J, Bonaccio M, Vitaglione P, Grosso G. Ultra-processed foods and nutritional dietary profile: a meta-analysis of nationally representative samples. *Nutrients*. 2021;13(10):3390. doi:10.3390/nu13103390

5. What You Need to Know about Processed Foods. UCLA Health. December 21, 2021. https://www.uclahealth.org/news/what-you-need-to-know-about-processed-foods-and-why-it-is-so-hard-to-quit-them

Chapter 10

The Temptation of Time and Convenience

Today, convenience is an overwhelming need and temptation. This has evolved for many reasons, such as mothers having to work full time (before 1980, more Moms stayed at home and had more time for cooking) and an increase in employees working overtime. There is also a large increase in people who are working multiple jobs to meet their financial needs.

What is my point here? My point is that people are tired. A Mom or Dad may get home from work and have three, or maybe four hours until the children go to bed. In those three or four hours, dinner has to be cooked and the kitchen has to be cleaned. It takes at least a half hour to prepare a decent home-cooked meal if you have all the ingredients that you need. You may even have to stop at a grocery store if you need certain items for dinner. Then, there may be one or two hours of homework and studying. Making quick choices at fast-food restaurants is the only answer for many. It's convenient, but it is also contributing to the obesity problem among Americans.

What You Can Do

Take baby steps: plan one night a week to slow down and make healthier choices for where you eat and what you choose to eat. Also, plan one night to eat at home and not cook frozen food. Actually cook a meal: grilled chicken, baked potatoes and a vegetable, pasta and homemade meatballs, or rice and pork chops with a vegetable. With Google allowing you to pull up any recipe, for any food, with detailed instructions and even videos on how to prepare it, no one can use the excuse that they don't know how to cook. After planning a healthy meal once a week, and a carefully selected healthier fast-food dinner one night a week, then try to do both twice a week. So, for two nights you will have a healthy home-cooked meal, and for two nights you will eat healthy fast food. Just make careful selections. Try this for a while and after some time, it should be easy for you to incorporate healthy eating into the other three nights. It will start to become a habit. You will start to become consciously aware of what you are eating for your meals and how you feel after you eat. It all is a process of slowing down and tuning in.

Does Homework Play A Role in Weight Gain/Obesity?

The "No Child Left Behind Act" of 2001 required states to develop assessments in basic skills. To receive funding, the schools must distribute these assessments to all students at select grade levels. The act was very controversial and was stripped of its national features in 2015 and replaced with the "Every Student Succeeds Act," returning power to the states. I bring attention to this act because one effect that it had on students, in my opinion, is that it required much more study time. Some students had other tests like college entrance exams to study for as well. Extra homework and studying drastically increased before testing so that the students could pass the tests and the schools could receive the anticipated funding. There was a time when teachers would spend months on a certain math concept. However, when trying to pass a test and you do not know what is going to be on the test, it makes sense to cover a lot more or all of the material. My kids definitely rolled through concepts faster than I remember doing in school. Trying to cover so much material in a short time can be frustrating—all in an effort to cover more material to pass the required assessments and then pass the tests. If you cover 10 concepts in a year, you may have 10 tests and let's just say 50 homework assignments. However, if you cover 20 concepts, you may have 20 tests and 100 homework assignments! How much has the curriculum changed to meet the required testing? How much has homework and test-taking increased? Is it too much?

Initiatives were created to promote exercise, requesting that all kids try to achieve 60 minutes of play or exercise per day. Was this because of the obesity problem or lack of exercise due to no time to exercise? This is a spectacular idea, however, with so much homework and studying to do now, the goal of 60 minutes of daily play may not always be possible.

Being Overly Busy

A child who wakes up fresh on a Saturday may get two hours of homework done in two hours. On the other hand, two hours of homework after a seven-hour day at school may take three or four hours because of their exhausted brain. Well-needed breaks and snacks in between getting loads of homework done can drag out the task, often becoming an all-evening event. The kids are tired and trying to complete all homework as swiftly as possible, to make time for play or exercise can be impractical. Hygiene, dinner, and after-school activities take up some evenings as well. With such a rigorous schedule and mounds of homework, a parent can feel bad putting more demands on their child to get 60 minutes of exercise, help cook dinner, or help with dishes after dinner.

Here is what happens: Frozen pizzas, frozen chicken nuggets on paper plates, or fast food and homework in the car on the way to extra-curricular activities, such as religion classes, tutoring, dance, or sports. Quick showers and what spare time is left is spent on computer games or electronics, before bed, because after making your child do everything he or she has to do in the evening for school, you feel compelled to give them the last bit of time to choose an activity that they really want to do. Let's face it, after a busy day, most kids choose the television, computer, or electronic games because they require the least energy. If your child is in an organized sport, then they may have achieved their 60 minutes of exercise. Kids' schedules today are very busy, much different from kids' schedules in the last century.

I Remember Those Days

I often think of how I worked 30 hours in my twenties and went to college in the evenings. It took me more than four years to finish college and when I was on the home stretch, I contemplated continuing for a master's degree and quickly decided NO WAY. I was so tired from working and going to school for years that I just wanted some time to myself. Currently, kids in middle and high school keep a very similar schedule to what mine was like in my twenties. They keep very busy in school during the day and in the evening as well. It doesn't surprise me that when they get a day when they have nothing to do, they do nothing!

On-the-Go and Convenience Eating

A busy schedule goes hand in hand with on-the-go eating. This is the time in your life when you realize how far away from the school your home is! Or, how far away from home your workplace is! Wouldn't it be great to live within 5 or 10 minutes of where you need to go daily? Sports, for some kids, currently, take up more time than they did 50 to 60 years ago. There are a lot of additional requirements, such as special practices, clinics, conditioning, and, of course, travel teams, many of which require overnight travel to different States.

Run, run, run, and no time for home-cooked meals. So, what is the result? We have talked about how fast food, convenience stores, and vending machines have all expanded and increased their selection and some stay open 24 hours a day. Food-delivery services are also much more available, meaning we can eat away from home as often as we want and at any time. Are we lucky that we can eat whenever and wherever we want? If you are concerned about the quality of the food that you are eating, then the answer is NO. Keep in mind that most processed and packaged foods and fast foods have higher salt, fat, and sugar than when you cook a meal at home or make food from home to go. On-the-go eating causes you to consume more calories.

Spending Time with School-Age Children

Whether you have a child with extra needs or not, in today's world, giving your kids your time can be one of the hardest things to give! Parents used to enjoy time alone. Remember this one? "Go outside and don't come in until the streetlights come on." Well, that was a popular saying a long time ago but now parents might be more apprehensive to send their kids outside for hours alone. Although it provided much exercise and exploratory value, it may not be considered safe today.

Today, with many moms working full time and squeezing in the must-dos, such as grocery shopping and helping with homework, coming up with a new game to play with your kids at 6.30 pm can be a hard task because you are exhausted. It is really tempting and very easy to offer up the T.V. or an electronic game. I admit that I took that route occasionally, but I think that in the back of our brains, we all know that it is not the healthiest choice. Some electronic games and computer games will captivate your little ones for hours, but it is well known that a sedentary lifestyle is unhealthy. In the final chapter of this book, I will share with you some of the most creative games and fun ideas that we created when our kids were little to keep them moving. It will introduce you to some non-standard uses of toys and furniture that make kids laugh and have a good time. Time is a challenge when you, as the parent, must think of the idea or game to play, do the preparations to set up the game, and then play the game as well.

After reading the list of games/ideas in this book, you can decide upon a game to play and possibly do the preparations the day before, or during your lunch hour, and this will eliminate a large part of the time it takes to kick the activities into motion! In addition to playing with your children, you will see that you will be teaching them about real life by incorporating this type of play into their young lives. For example, they can learn about the profession of a chef, office worker, store owner, schoolteacher, daycare attendant, nurse or doctor, professional athlete, chemist, etc. Your time and effort may help your child someday choose what they want to be when they grow up. Your efforts will inspire creativity in your child and provide a secure sense that they have a parent or parents who care and love them very much.

Special Note to the "Runners"

There is time if you make it, so take charge. When my kids were in school, many families seemed to be doing twelve things in one weekend. They seemed to enjoy telling you what they were doing and where they were going. I have always been one to NOT jump on the bandwagon. Spending time with your kids does not have to involve buying tickets, traveling by car, or enrolling them in classes or sports. And you take them there and wait for them. Occasionally, they need time to have nothing to do but hang out with you. They need their parents to be with them but not on the phone, driving the car, or dropping them off. Some parents have been "going non-stop" for so long that they may not know how to slow down. Not to mention, "running"—always being on the go—is a large reason for the fast-food dinners that aren't the healthiest choice. There is nothing wrong with creating your own fun, but society today compels us to think that we have to check off stereotypical "to-dos" on a parenting bucket list that usually involves going places and spending money.

Teenagers who may not want to play games can be more of a challenge to get moving. If this is your scenario, then the "Post Organized Sports" chapter in this book may be helpful to you.

Chapter 11

Are Food Additives Making Us Fat?

Before beginning to read, please note that the information in this chapter is subject to change as additives in food, policies, and laws change over time. This information is included to provide a basic understanding of this dynamic field.

A friend of mine, who is overweight, asked me during lunch one day if I was going to include a chapter in this book about how the food industry is putting ingredients in food products that are causing obesity. I said, "Of course," but I really didn't have any information on this issue. Up until that point, I had never researched the modern-day practice of adding chemicals to our food, such as antibiotics and trans-fats—which have now been largely banned from the food market—and many other additives. However, it was not the first time that someone asked me if modern food additives are the reason for the widespread obesity documented in the U.S., so I decided to write this chapter.

My experience

My first thought after being asked this question was, "Why hasn't this process affected me yet?" Please understand that I do not have any specific information on whether food chemicals, preservatives, or additives lead to weight gain, but this is what I noticed through my own experience. When a possible gluten allergy emerged in our household, I began purchasing gluten-free products. Many of these products came from Italy, and I noticed the pureness of the products compared to the non-gluten-free products I previously used. The products from Italy did not have extra additives or preservatives. I wondered if the allergy was really to gluten or possibly to the additives and preservatives that were in the products that we had been consuming. I noticed that the number of colds, allergy attacks, and infections in our family seemed to decrease as we ate a better diet that was free of these additives. This is when I realized the importance of flipping food packages over to see what ingredients were in the product. Also, I need to mention that I do not eat a lot of ultra-processed food and I am not overweight. I do not know if those two facts are related to each other. However, if you don't really know what an ingredient is and there is not much research on this ingredient, in my opinion, it is best to avoid it or at least, limit your intake until proper research can be completed.

Researching

The NCBI's (National Center for Biotechnology Information) core literature database is called PubMed® (https://pubmed.ncbi.nlm.nih.gov/) which provides abstracts and citations for millions of articles from thousands of biomedical journals. The highly technical PubMed® includes more than 37 million citations of work published in the biomedical literature from MEDLINE, life science journals, and online books. Citations may include additional links to full-text content from PubMed Central and publisher websites. It would be quite an undertaking to try and review all food additives that you may find listed on the packaging of foods that you are purchasing and I certainly have not attempted this task but below is some notable information.

Among the articles compiled by PubMed is a recent review by Pearlman and colleagues entitled "The Association Between Artificial Sweeteners and Obesity" with the following information:

> Although artificial sweeteners were developed as a sugar substitute to help reduce insulin resistance and obesity, data in both animal models and humans suggest that the effects of artificial sweeteners may contribute to metabolic syndrome and the obesity epidemic. Artificial sweeteners appear to change the host microbiome, lead to decreased satiety, and alter glucose homeostasis, and are associated with increased caloric consumption and weight gain. [1]

Similar reviews discussed the impact of sugar-sweetened beverages on weight gain[2] and the metabolic effects of artificial sweeteners in young persons.[3] An eye-opening review written by Ravichandran and colleagues[4] entitled "Food Obesogens As Emerging Metabolic Disruptors: a Toxicological Insight" explained that there are about more than 10,000 chemicals allowed in food largely due to weak enforcement and that regulatory bodies are tasked with identifying chemicals that are inadequately tested or not tested at all for safety. In addition, in his review of the epidemic of obesity and its relationship to changes in food intake, Bray noted that the rise in HFCS intake paralleled the increased prevalence of obesity.[5]

Although the results are currently far from clear, there appears to be some data confirming the negative effects of numerous food additives. Further research will be needed to understand the potential effects of food additives on weight gain. However, as stated earlier, there are many additives to consider and it will take a lot of work and time to explore and confirm these results. However, in the meantime, avoidance would be a good idea in my opinion.

Other speculations on the internet suggest that food additives might contribute to disorders ranging from nausea, asthma, hyperactivity, cancer, headaches, mood disturbances, reduced mental performance, leukemia, gastrointestinal cancer, and brain tumors.

Many people do not even realize that food products have additives in them as they are not in the habit of flipping over a food package to see what exactly they are consuming.

GMO (genetically modified organisms) and "bioengineered" food ingredients

Among the 10,000 food additives in the United States, you may see the term GMO (genetically modified organism, such as a plant, animal, microorganism, or other organism).[6] This term is being replaced in the United States food marketplace by the term "Bioengineered". Bioengineered food ingredients contain genetic material that has been modified through laboratory techniques and for which the modification could not be obtained through conventional breeding or found naturally. Beginning in 2022, retail food products containing or produced with the help of GMOs were required to be labeled as such in words, a symbol, or links that convey the information thus making the products more detectable to the public.

Are GMO and Bioengineered foods safe?

The U.S. Food and Drug Administration (FDA), U.S. Environmental Protection Agency (EPA), and U.S. Department of Agriculture (USDA) are responsible for ensuring that GMOs are safe for human, plant, and animal health.[7,8] However, there is some opposition to Bioengineered

Foods and GMO foods debating that there is a lack of proper regulation and unbiased scientific research on their long-term impact on human and environmental health. Further research will be needed to ensure the safety of these products. In the meantime, if you are skeptical, here are a few ways to avoid these foods:

How to avoid GMOs/Bioengineered foods

1. Buy food that is labeled 100 percent organic with no GMOs - many organic foods have a non-GMO or GMO-free label/symbol.
2. Choose organic whole foods that you can prepare yourself instead of processed or prepackaged foods.
3. Purchase grass-fed beef.
4. Purchase products at local farmers' markets.

Trans Fat

This additive was added to processed foods to increase shelf life for 30 to 40 years. The FDA has, since November 2013, banned trans fats from the United States food market. The removal process is a slow and continuous effort, and it may take some time to achieve complete elimination.

Trans fats are one of the unhealthiest additives, mainly because they cause cholesterol problems. Trans fats, or partially hydrogenated oils, are found in deep-fried foods, baked goods, margarine, and vegetable shortening. This additive is under suspicion for increasing the risk of heart disease and Type 2 diabetes. Most researchers agree that eating trans fats can be harmful to your health because it lowers good cholesterol (HDL) and raises bad cholesterol (LDL).

The American Heart Association recommends getting less than 1% of your daily calories from trans fats. Trans fats may be in foods sold in many restaurants and usually, that means no nutrition labels, thus making it hard to see how much trans-fat you have just consumed. A good rule to follow is usually when you increase your consumption of processed foods, you increase trans fats as well. Hopefully, the ban on trans fats has helped with reducing the amount in your diet.

Limit your intake!

For those concerned about weight gain, it is crucial to remember that if you consume large amounts of sugary or unhealthy, processed, high-fat foods frequently, you may gain weight just from the frequency and or large portion of the food item. Large portions can be a culprit of weight gain. Unhealthy high-fat foods and highly processed foods are sometimes eaten in abundance due to their convenience. Cooking a healthy meal at home is bypassed for a quick but unhealthy meal. Eating your entire daily intake of calories from unhealthy high-fat foods such as baked goods and fried foods, can contribute to weight gain. If you consume a lot of these foods, try reducing the amount by eating them once a day only, then once every other day, and then once a week, and so on until they are not a main part of your diet. By limiting these foods, you will start to notice a difference in how you feel, and it will be positive.

What YOU add - Condiment Crazy

The 2000s have been the age of food creation and decoration, not just for manufacturers but also for **self-induced sprinkling, dipping, shaking, and squirting.** Sugar, fat, and salt can also be added to foods by YOU, and that can cause weight gain as well. Be cautious of how much sugar and cream you add to your coffee, be careful how much mayonnaise or butter you spread on your bread, how much chocolate syrup you add to your ice cream, and how much dressing you add to your salad. Not adding or reducing the amount you add can help you avoid gaining weight.

Adding Sugar

There was a time when vanilla or chocolate ice cream was just enough, no toppings needed. Vanilla pudding and yogurt were sweet enough without extra toppings. People didn't add lots of cream and sweetener to their plain black coffee. Considering the calories of every self-induced sprinkle, dip, shake, squirt, top, and pour might surprise you. These additions are not free—they count toward your daily calorie intake!

Adding Fat

Breaded, fried, coated, dipped, battered, sautéed, crispy, sizzled, smothered, drizzled, loaded, stuffed, layered, and melted are all extra actions! Extra dressing, extra cheese, extra butter and sour cream, and extra ranch dressing are all additions that you choose! These are not terms that were used often or at all at the beginning of the last century.

When I was a child and would visit my grandparents, I would often see their dinner on the stove, which was a casserole dish with meat, potatoes, and vegetables in it and maybe a little oil—and nothing else!

Salt - We May Assume It Is Natural - Too Much of Anything Is No Good

The American Heart Association recommends no more than 2,300 milligrams (mg) of sodium a day and moving toward an ideal limit of no more than 1,500 mg per day for most adults. On average, most Americans eat more than 3,400 mg of sodium each day, much more than the American Heart Association and other health organizations recommend.

High salt products

Why do Americans eat so much salt? Well, 70% of the sodium Americans consume comes from packaged, prepared, and restaurant foods, not the saltshaker. Eating a lot of salt can cause your body to retain more water, which can show up on the scale as extra pounds and leave you feeling like a walking human swimming pool. You might be surprised at how much extra water weight you can hold! Also, high-salt diets appear to be linked to higher body fat[9]—in particular, the kind of fat that accumulates around your middle. Not to mention, too much salt in your diet can contribute to hypertension, one of the leading risk factors for cardiovascular disease. Checking the salt per serving size on packaged, frozen, and prepared foods is an easy way to start monitoring some of your daily salt intake. This will provide an idea of how much salt you are consuming in contrast with what your recommended intake should be – you may be surprised!

Salt Can Make You Thirsty

Having a child with diabetes can be very tough on sick days when insulin is on board but due to influenza or a cold, hunger is absent. This can be very scary, but I learned a helpful trick. Providing salty snacks made my daughter thirsty so she would then drink a sugary drink which would keep her blood sugar from going too low due to not eating much. If you prefer sugary drinks over water and you are eating salty foods your thirst may be amplified by the salt, making you want to drink more to quench your thirst and thus take in more sugar.

Dull Taste Sense

I was cooking with a friend once, who is older than I am, and he asked me for the salt. I gave him my saltshaker. He was shaking rapidly and then looked at me and said, "Give me the salt!" and he made his hands show a bigger size. I realized that he wanted the salt container that I use to fill my little saltshaker—the one with the silver pour spout! This made me wonder why some people need or want so much salt. It could be what they are accustomed to, perhaps it's the way they have been eating for years. If you frequently eat high salt, there is a chance that your taste buds are just acclimated to a high amount of salt, or you may have dull or damaged taste buds.

> **Some possible reasons why taste buds become dull:**
>
> • Sinus problems
>
> • A head injury that might affect the nerves related to taste and smell
>
> • Dental problems that can release a bad taste into your mouth
>
> • Age
>
> • Medication
>
> • Illness
>
> • Cancer treatment
>
> • Smoking

If you think calories are hard to count, trying to count sodium will probably blow your mind—it isn't easy! Some fast-food items have their nutrition facts online so you can check to see what the salt content is. **However, here are some tips:**

1. Remember that the American Heart Association recommends no more than **2,300** milligrams (mg) of sodium a day and **moving toward an ideal limit of no more than 1,500 mg.** When eating packaged food, check the sodium content. Look at the menu to see sodium content. Set a goal to keep your sodium intake under 2,300 mg.

2. The best way to limit your salt consumption is to **eat fresh and minimally processed foods found around the perimeter of the**

store. Fruits, vegetables, whole grains, legumes (beans), nuts, plant-based protein, lean animal protein and fish. Eating these foods will help you with limiting your salt/sodium intake if you do not add additional salt.

3. **Don't shake too much!** Or worse yet, don't take the lid off the saltshaker to dump or dip a spoon in to get a mound of salt to add to your food. My personal trick is to keep the saltshaker in the spice cabinet during cooking and it usually remains there for dinner. I may take it out for a few shakes during cooking, but then I put it back.

4. **Not all saltshakers are equal**. Make sure you don't have a fire-hose saltshaker and if you do, throw it out and buy one that doesn't "dump" salt out. Salt is meant to be lightly sprinkled.

5. **Eliminating or reducing your intake of frozen, fast foods and fried foods** will reduce your salt intake. There is a lot of sodium in fast food because salt acts as a preservative. Also, salt adds flavor and it can make certain foods easier to process, thus making it a very helpful ingredient for some food manufacturers.

6. **Don't combine super-salty items**. Just like we spoke about with high-fat and high-sugar foods, do not combine salty items with other salty items like pretzels and pepperoni or hotdogs and potato chips. Too many salty foods together are going to be bad for you over time.

7. **When cooking,** take into account that many canned goods and some spice blends may already contain a high salt content, so you do not need to add as much from the salt shaker while cooking or before eating.

8. **Taste your food BEFORE you add salt**. Pay attention to your food when you eat it to determine if it needs salt. Try to go without adding salt. Look at the label and see how much salt/sodium it already has.

Avoid Too Much Added Salt in Food, But Do Drink a Lot of Water

Benefits of Drinking Water

The human body needs water. Staying hydrated is vital for health and well-being. Water is a great replacement for sugary drinks and can reduce your daily carbs and calories drastically. For example, 16 oz (240 ml) of a well-known brand of soda contains 27 g total carbs, 27 g net carbs, 0g fat, 0g protein, and 100 calories. If you have three of these sodas per day that is 300 extra calories, or if you are counting carbs, an extra 81 g of carbs. This soda contains zero fat and protein and has very little nutritional value if any. Water and a healthy food item containing 300 calories and nutrients would be a much better choice.

Water consumption is important because adult humans are made up of 60% water, and blood plasma is 90% water. All the cells and organs of the body need water to function properly. Water forms the basis of blood, digestive juices, urine, and perspiration, and is contained in lean muscle, fat, and bones. The body can't store water, so we need to replenish our supply every day to make up for losses through the lungs, skin, urine, and feces. Your body loses water every time you breathe. You lose about 1 cup of water each day, just from breathing! A dry mouth and lips may be a sign that you need a glass of water!

Here Are Some Reasons Our Body Needs Water:

- It delivers oxygen through the body.
- Water is essential for the kidneys, and it prevents kidney damage.
- It flushes body waste.
- It helps maintain blood pressure.
- It makes minerals and nutrients accessible.
- Your airways need water and a lack of it can make asthma and allergies worse.
- It regulates body temperature.
- It lubricates the joints—and helps you avoid joint pain.
- It forms saliva and mucus which helps with digestion and keeping the mouth, nose, and eyes moist and prevents tooth decay.

- It cushions the brain, spinal cord, and other sensitive tissues.
- It boosts skin health and beauty.
- When dehydrated, the skin can become more vulnerable to skin disorders and wrinkling.
- The digestive system depends on it and a lack of water can lead to constipation, heartburn, and stomach ulcers.
- It boosts performance during exercise.

As you can see, drinking water instead of sugary drinks may help with weight loss and a whole lot more benefits besides! If you do not like the taste of water, try adding citrus fruit (lemons, limes, oranges) to make the water taste better. You can add a teaspoon of natural sugar to your water, which contains a mere 16 calories, and put it in a shaker with ice. You will be surprised how delicious it can taste. By replacing soda with water, you will be avoiding chemicals, calories, and carbs and taking major steps toward improving your health.

There is no universally agreed quantity of water that must be consumed daily, so start off slowly and do the best that you can. Remember, every 16 oz soda that you replace with water can reduce your daily calories by possibly 100!

The Bottom Line: Avoidance May Help Prevent Weight Gain and Disease

I believe the reason I am not gaining weight from food additives is that I am not a big consumer of high-fructose corn syrup, unhealthy, processed high-fat, high-salt, and high-sugar items - at least, not on a consistent basis. I avoid dessert and rarely eat baked goods, margarine, and vegetable shortening. I do not eat a lot of processed, ultra-processed, and packaged foods. I avoid frozen foods and convenience store eating. I am not a big consumer of products with trans fats. I am salt/sodium conscious and try to avoid foods and spices that contain a high salt content or are heavily salted. I do not own a deep fryer and I don't order deep-fried foods when I am out. I recognize the basic diet of only eating breakfast, lunch, and dinner with small healthy snacks possibly in between. I have portion control and rarely overeat. I avoid fast food and choose good-quality restaurants with healthy options. I am cautious of how many condiments I add to my food and I drink a lot of water. On occasion I do eat unhealthy foods, no one is perfect, but I try very hard to eat healthy daily.

For this reason, I have not been affected by food additives thus far. Due to my familiarity with diabetes, I was fortunate to learn how to pay more attention to foods, their labels, and what kind of effect they can have on the human body. Someone who does not need to pay attention to foods and their effects as I do may be unaware of this information, and being unaware could result in food additives and additions playing a big part in weight gain. The simple answer, for now, is they can't affect you if you don't eat them.

A "high-quality diet" does not include a daily dose of unhealthy processed foods. Whether you add or it is served to you, sugar and unhealthy processed high-fat foods are not good consistently. A quality diet does not include excessive deep-fried foods, baked goods, margarine, vegetable shortening, or ultra-processed foods. Eating these foods daily will potentially make you gain weight!

Final thoughts

It is easy to say that we should just not buy these products, but considering that more and more additives are being utilized, that might be nearly impossible. No one really knows, yet, if these additives in our food ingredients are causing weight gain or disease. However, if these ingredients have a negative effect or are not being properly absorbed (we are not sure yet) and not counting as nutrition then we could be depleting ourselves of nutrients. The last time America had a nutrition problem, and disease was abundant, was in the early part of the last century, as mentioned earlier, and it was addressed with food fortification or adding vitamins to correct many diseases. If America is having an increase in diseases in the 2000s, it may be due, once again, to poor nutrition. Not because of what our food is lacking but maybe because of what is in our food that may not be healthy or may be unable to be absorbed properly. This is a question I ponder and only time will tell. The 1940s to the 1990s, in my opinion, were some of the best years for healthy food manufacturing and consumption and many of us are not eating the simple foods of the early part of the last century.

But in doing the research for this chapter, I discovered another interesting point, which is that maybe it is not so much what they are putting into our food, but, rather, what is **NOT** in our food, what is missing in our food. See the Chapter on Complex and Simple Carbohydrates.

Literature Cited in this Chapter

1. Pearlman M, Obert J, Casey L. The association between artificial sweeteners and obesity. *Current Gastroenterology Reports*. 2017;19(12). doi:10.1007/s11894-017-0602-9

2. Malik VS, Schulze MB, Hu FB. Intake of sugar-sweetened beverages and weight gain: a systematic review. *The American Journal of Clinical Nutrition*. 2006;84(2):274-288. doi:10.1093/ajcn/84.1.274

3. Brown RJ, De Banate MA, Rother KI. Artificial Sweeteners: A systematic review of metabolic effects in youth. *International Journal of Pediatric Obesity*. 2010;5(4):305-312. doi:10.3109/17477160903497027

4. Ravichandran G, Lakshmanan DK, Arunachalam A, Thilagar S. Food obesogens as emerging metabolic disruptors; A toxicological insight. *Journal of Steroid Biochemistry and Molecular Biology.* 2022;217:106042. doi:10.1016/j.jsbmb.2021.106042

5. Bray GA. The epidemic of obesity and changes in food intake: the Fluoride Hypothesis. *Physiology & Behavior*. 2004;82(1):115-121. doi:10.1016/j.physbeh.2004.04.033

6. Murray M. GMOs and Bioengineered Food Labeling: What You Need to Know. May 2023. https://www.iherb.com/blog/what-is-non-gmo/239

7. United States Department of Agriculture. What is Bioengineered Food? https://www.ams.usda.gov/sites/default/files/media/BE_Consumer.pdf

8. United States Food and Drug Administration. How GMOs are Regulated in the United States. March 5, 2024. https://www.fda.gov/food/agricultural-biotechnology/how-gmos-are-regulated-united-states

9. Zhang X, Wang J, Li J, Yu Y, Song Y. A positive association between dietary sodium intake and obesity and central obesity: results from the National Health and Nutrition Examination Survey 1999-2006. *Nutrition Research*. 2018;55:33-44. doi:10.1016/j.nutres.2018.04.008

Chapter 12

Be Smarter – Complex and Simple Carbohydrates

Despite what some diets tell you, your body needs carbohydrates. They are important for your body's inner workings as they provide energy. When we eat carbs, our digestive system breaks them down into glucose, which is what our cells need for fuel. If glucose is in short supply, then your body looks elsewhere—like your muscle tissue and can actually start to break down your muscle tissue.

Carbohydrates are made up of fiber, starch, and sugar. Fiber and starch are **complex carbs** while sugar is a **simple carb**.

Simple carbs are sugars, such as glucose, fructose, and sucrose; while some sugars occur in foods naturally, most sugar in the American diet is *added* sugar, for example, high-fructose corn syrup. To make it easy to understand, whole or complex carbohydrates are a better choice for your health than simple carbohydrates. Complex carbs contain fiber and are generally unrefined/unprocessed: fruits and vegetables, wholewheat bread, beans, wholegrain cereal, corn, oats, peas, and rice.

Simple carbs are not as healthy as complex carbs. Examples of simple carbs are candy, sugary drinks, syrups, table sugar, fruit juice concentrate, and products with added sugar such as baked goods and some cereals. Refined grains also have a similar effect on the body to simple carbs because they've had all the fiber removed. When grains are processed, they are stripped of their fiber and nutrients and so act like sugar in the body. Complex carbs are in their original state and contain fiber and nutrients—and therefore they're digested more slowly.

Simple carbs are digested quickly and broken down to glucose— which is rapidly absorbed into the bloodstream. Why is this bad for our health? Visualize this: A child pours a 10-pound bag of sugar into a 5-pound canister and they pour slowly to just fill to the top. Then an avalanche happens and the sugar pours out way too fast and overflows down the sides. When we eat simple carbs in large portions, our body is overwhelmed, and it stores some of the glucose as FAT. Just as the sugar spills over the sides of the container, you will spill over your jeans. However, when you eat complex carbs, the pouring process is much more controlled, as if an adult was pouring very slowly and making sure the sugar doesn't spill over the top. There is no mess or overflow to take care of afterward! A slow pour = slow digestion, meaning slower absorption of glucose into the body.

If you continue to eat simple carbs in large amounts, your body will keep storing some as fat. Plus, if you don't exercise, the fat is never burned and so it builds and builds around your waist leading to a large belly.

The fiber in complex carbs also makes you feel fuller for longer because they are digested more slowly. Therefore, you may desire less food. It takes more energy to digest a complex carb. Simple carbs are rapidly digested, leaving you hungry sooner.

If complex carbs are not in your daily diet, you are missing a high-quality fiber-containing nutrient.

Chapter 13

High Sugar in Food, Unhealthy High Fat – a Deadly Combination

Sugar is everywhere, more so than ever before. High-sugar drinks such as smoothies, milkshakes, soda, and sweet coffees are among the most popular ways to get your "sugar fix." You can get these drinks in malls, fast food restaurants, shopping plazas, convenience stores, gas stations, hotels, etc. Whatever you want, you won't have too much trouble finding it. However, if you have diabetes, or pre-diabetes, or if you are on a diet, you may be having a hard time as a sugar addict. Why? It is because of the "roller coaster" or "swing" effect that high sugar content can cause. If you are trying to manage diabetes or have success with a diet, keeping your sugar intake as consistent as possible will help. What do I mean by consistent? Having too much sugar obviously will make you gain weight but sugar, also, is very hard on your pancreas, blood sugar, and energy stability. If you have diabetes, high sugar content can raise your blood sugar super high and then possibly drop your blood sugar very quickly. It can also cause your blood sugar to remain high, depending on what you have had to eat earlier and how active you are after consuming it. Someone who does not have diabetes, may experience an energy boost and then an energy crash and a feeling of fatigue.

Some people substitute a large coffee drink for a meal. They order non-fat milk or skim milk thinking that this is a good idea to reduce calories. However, compared to the amount of carbohydrates the drink contains, the fat/protein is very low. Fat and protein can help slow the absorption of glucose into the blood. This means this high-sugar drink can quickly spike blood sugar, especially if you order extra pumps of syrup! This can also rob you of energy hours later when your blood sugar crashes and you may experience extreme hunger as well.

The "Roller Coaster" Effect

Here is what the "roller coaster" effect may do for both insulin-dependent and non-insulin dependent people. When my daughter was a child, I took her out to eat dinner one night. She gave herself a shot before leaving. She was in the normal range (100–150). After ordering the food, the server brought her a soda and my daughter drank the soda while waiting for her food. The food was taking a while and the server, without asking, brought her another soda. I suggested not drinking it, but she took a few sips anyway. Soda typically has very high sugar content. I have learned, over the years that a drink with 15 to 20 grams of sugar seems to work well for our particular case of diabetes management. A soda drink may contain 35 to 55 grams of sugar or more. After drinking the soda, her blood sugar rapidly escalated and by the time her dinner arrived, she was not very hungry. Why? When her blood sugar rises quickly, she doesn't feel hungry anymore. She feels jittery, and she feels like she needs to stop eating and drinking to avoid feeling worse. In this situation, for a someone without diabetes, of course, your blood sugar will not rise so high, but your pancreas will have to work very, very hard to keep your blood sugar low. Years and years of abusing your pancreas (making it work very hard by consuming high-sugar foods) will exhaust it and eventually, it may give up—and at that point, you may acquire pre-diabetes. My daughter did not eat too much of her dinner and I knew that she had just climbed the first hill on that roller coaster. I knew that she would plummet in a couple of hours (due to lack of food). How much protein and fat she had earlier in the day and how active she would be after dinner would determine how soon her blood sugar would plummet. If she had consumed her dinner with the soda, her blood sugar may have never risen (if enough insulin had been given). Or if there wasn't enough insulin, her sugar may have risen to require a bit more insulin but the chances of a plummet in blood sugar would be less because she would at least have had fat and protein from dinner on board. But since she hardly ate, she had nothing in her system to "hold" the blood sugar or keep it from nose-diving. Basically, the blood sugar went sky-high and had no safety net (fat and protein) to ease the drop. I'll provide a couple of examples.

If my daughter had a protein-and-fat-packed lunch, fried chicken sandwich, and French fries and then had the 2 sodas for dinner, her blood sugar would have spiked to a very high number and then possibly stayed high due to the high protein and fat at lunch still releasing and "holding" the blood sugar. If she had a very light lunch (salad) and then had the two sodas she may have spiked to a high number at dinner, and then she would have plummeted due to not having a lot of protein or fat from the lunchtime salad that would "hold" her blood sugar and keep it from dropping very fast. The KEY is to have a medium amount of your daily recommended fat and protein with every meal to avoid spikes and plummets. Eating foods high in sugar spikes blood sugar and eating high fat helps that spike stay high. Eating foods with high sugar and high fat together OR separately is not good for consistency with your blood sugar. This may sound complicated to you, but it really is not. I can sum it up easily for you by saying, as I did at the beginning of this book, consistency is key to maintaining good blood sugar and having success with a diet. Consuming super high-sugar foods, super unhealthy high fat, and protein **inconsistently** will make it very hard for a someone with diabetes to maintain "in range" numbers. For someone without diabetes, it will cause "swings" in your energy and desire to eat. You may feel full for a long time and then feel famished and eat more than you should to suppress your extreme feeling of hunger or fatigue. If you do not have diabetes, but your pancreas is working extremely hard, you may feel tired or have fatigue.

Others Weigh In On the Impact of Fat on Blood Sugar

A recent study published in the *European Journal of Nutrition* found that diets high in fat, and in saturated fat in particular, resulted in increased insulin resistance.[1] While increases in abdominal fat can contribute to poor insulin health, dietary fat seems to affect insulin resistance even in people who are weight stable and don't see increases in their abdominal fat levels, according to the researchers. This finding was discussed at length in an article published in EveryDay Health.[2]

High-fat foods are okay in moderation—after all, as part of a balanced meal, healthy fats from foods such as nuts, avocados, and salmon can slow the release of glucose into the bloodstream. Current federal guidelines recommend that about 20 to 35% of your daily calories come from fat and that saturated fat from foods such as cheese, red meat, fried foods, and baked goods should make up less than 10% of your daily caloric intake.

Another article from WebMD.com, entitled "20 Reasons for Blood Sugar Swings" also agrees[3].

> When you dig into a plate of sesame beef or sweet and sour chicken, it isn't just the white rice that can cause a problem.

High-fat foods can make your blood sugar stay up for longer. The same is true for pizza, French fries, and other goodies that have a lot of carbs and fat.

What is not mentioned here is that when fat and protein are not on board but there is a high sugar content in the food/drink, an avalanche can happen.

The Avalanche!

After being home for a couple of hours, my daughter checked her blood sugar, and she was still in a high range (220) from the soda. But, having done this for years, I knew the landslide was coming. Foods that contain high sugar are "mean" to your body. In less than a half-hour, her mood changed, and I could see she was getting edgy, I knew that she needed to eat soon. As I was making something for her to eat, I asked her to check her finger once again, and she was 45. The drop was so sudden—from 220 to 45 in a half-hour. Keep in mind activity level also plays a role in how fast blood sugar may drop. This is what high sugar content without fat or protein can do. This is the danger of high sugar content and what it does to your body. After someone who takes insulin has plummeted, they may feel that they can't get enough juice/food to feel better. For someone who is not insulin-dependent, it is the same: after eating a lot of sugar you may feel full for a while but then in an hour or so you may feel famished and overeat to try to make yourself feel better. This is hard on your pancreas. This "roller coaster" effect also contributes to mood swings. My daughter describes rising and dropping quickly as a feeling you don't want to have. Jittery, anxious, shaky, confused, and even sick are some words that she uses to explain to me what she is feeling. When she eats properly and avoids very sugary foods and unhealthy high-fat foods, she seems to feel much better. For over a decade, I tried to keep my daughter away from high sugar content foods and unhealthy high fat and believe me, it was not easy. Our society loves these foods, and they are just about EVERYWHERE. Many people do not also realize the importance of what you ate earlier. I agree this part of diabetes is somewhat complicated when you first learn about it. But, if you are successful with understanding it, your blood sugar management will improve. This is equally important for someone who is on a diet. An easy way to avoid swings in your blood sugar, hunger feelings, mood, and energy levels is to avoid foods with high sugar and unhealthy high fat content.

A More In-Depth Look for Those Who Want to Understand

How Fat, Protein, and Sugar Interact

Fat/protein can be very helpful for dieters and someone with diabetes but can also make dieting and diabetes very difficult when consuming unhealthy fats or very high protein that you do not prepare for. What do I mean by helpful? Well, for someone with diabetes, as mentioned previously, fat and protein can keep your blood sugar from dropping too fast and that is good. But too much of anything is not good and this definitely is true for fat. I mention protein here because often fat and protein can work in the same way when it comes to blood sugar. Healthy protein is great most of the time but if consumed in too large amounts or along with high fat it can keep blood sugar from dropping when it should. For example, I've noticed, through experience, that nuts hold blood sugar and prevent it from dropping when it should because they have a lot of protein and fat (and it's easy to eat more than the suggested serving size). For dieters, fat and protein can provide a full feeling longer and possibly aid in a more consistent energy level and mood. But if you are consuming a lot of protein alone, it may be just like unhealthy high fat and hold your blood sugar or even elevate it. This is why I mention protein in this chapter as well. A person using insulin takes insulin before they eat to keep their blood sugar in a good range and when they eat their blood sugar may elevate slightly but the insulin should bring it back down. So, when I say high fat/protein may keep your blood sugar from dropping it means it stops the insulin from working or doing its job and more insulin may have to be given. For a person with diabetes, high sugar content or fat/protein, inconsistently, can interfere with insulin doing what it is expected to do. Insulin is pretty robotic and will usually do what it is expected to do; however, food choices can throw a disturbing wrench into the works. I saw my father, who had type 2, suffer from fluctuating numbers due to a fluctuating diet as well. It should be noted that other factors can disrupt insulin from doing its expected job, as well, such as stress and sickness.

I often compare a proper amount of good fat or protein to a coffee filter that slowly but easily holds coffee but also allows seepage perfectly (allowing sugar to drop). Unhealthy fats like French fries and too much protein can act as a canvas-type material, not allowing any seepage (blood sugar drop), and too little fat or protein can act as a Kleenex allowing too much seepage/total breakthrough (blood sugar drops way too fast). Diabetes can be very tricky, and consistency is key. Having that coffee filter (fat/protein - suggested daily amount) with every meal is best.

In My Opinion

Fat and protein calories have always been considered part of a balanced diet. Although carbs have the greatest effect on blood glucose, I have found fat and proteins (too many or none at all) also affect blood glucose control even when carbs are measured accurately. Some people utilizing the pump are taught only carbs are important, but I have found fat and protein to be very important especially if they fluctuate from day to day. It is like having a party and a few extra people show up or don't show up – no big deal. However, that one time when 20 extra people show up – it may become a problem. If most of the time your fat and protein range is with in recommended daily amounts (20–35% of total calories) but then one day you eat a very high-fat meal your blood sugar numbers may be affected. When fat is consumed in large quantities, it can raise blood sugar levels several hours later. The same can be true of protein. Meals that are high in protein content may cause blood sugar levels to rise several hours later—and may cause insulin-resistant blood sugar. So, for some people, protein and fat may impact blood glucose and insulin needs, depending on the quantity eaten, digestion, absorption, and composition of the meal. When my daughter was diagnosed, I was taught the importance of eating a balanced diet and how this would help her. Therefore, in my opinion, all three nutrients are important for people with diabetes.

For anyone trying to diet, you might have the general belief that you should stay away from sugar. If you ask someone who doesn't have diabetes what diabetes is, they may say that if you have diabetes, you cannot eat sugar. The word "sugar" is the word most often used when describing diabetes. If you ask someone who knows a little about diabetes you may hear the word "carbohydrates" or "carbs." If you acquire diabetes, you will learn that you must "count your carbs" and "watch your sugar intake." But you may not hear, as often, the word "fat" or "protein" associated with diabetes when talking about dietary needs for diabetes. The truth is fat/protein intake, especially high fat, is very important in dieting and diabetes control. The problem is many people do not realize this. You might be thinking, "Oh, no sugar, and now I have to worry about fat and protein too." Yes, you do! But it's not that hard. To make things very easy, just think of *the right amount of healthy fat and protein* as your "safety net." Anyone who has diabetes, (especially

Type 1), knows that you can "go low" or "drop" quickly. This means that you feel good and then all of a sudden you are shaky or lightheaded because of a drop in your blood sugar. Or, for someone who does not have diabetes you may feel good and then suddenly you are famished and need food quickly and the result is you overeat. Whenever I prepare a meal for myself or someone else, I consider if there is a healthy fat/protein that will be a "safety net" that will hold the blood sugar from dropping too fast (someone with diabetes) and keep someone without diabetes from the feeling of starving in a couple of hours. The carbs and the sugar raise blood sugar, give energy, and satisfy the feeling of hunger but it is the fat (and protein) that will sustain that satisfying feeling that will hold the blood sugar and keep it from dropping in a landslide fashion. Sugars and simple carbs are absorbed quickly after they are eaten. Fat and protein are absorbed very slowly. So, if you wake up and have a large coffee with lots of sugar but not much fat or protein in an hour and a half or two hours you will have no "safety net" there to hold your blood sugar or for someone without diabetes, the feeling of "starvation "will arise. For someone with diabetes, this is very dangerous. If one day you count your carbs for breakfast but have little or no fat, your results may be different if the next day you count the same carbs but have fat/protein as well with that meal. Why? Because the day that you eat fat/protein with your meal you will have that "safety net" that will slow or stop the drop in blood sugar. For someone without diabetes, the fat/protein will slow your feeling of being so hungry and or fatigued a couple of hours late.

My husband and I often shared the responsibility of checking my daughter's blood sugar late at night when she was sleeping. If he was checking, and I was going to sleep early, he would ask, "What is the fat?" I would tell him what she had for dinner and before bed but what was most important was the fat and protein—the safety net that would carry her through the night. If her blood sugar was low, and she didn't have a lot of fat/protein then she would be given orange juice with "whey powder" (protein) to raise her blood sugar and then hold it throughout the rest of the night. If her blood sugar was in a normal range, and she had a lot of fat and or protein before bed, she would most likely be fine and we would not expect her sugar to drop. (We could go to sleep!) If she was in good range but had "high fat" she would most likely rise. This latter scenario was the one that would cause us to stay up and recheck her blood sugar to see if we had to give insulin because her blood sugar would rise and stay high, and then we would have to recheck in a couple of hours.

Can fat and protein raise your blood sugar? In my opinion, yes, it can—this conclusion is based on my experience and articles I have read that agree with this point. It can cause inconsistency and create a roller coaster effect. Why do some say no? First of all, to make an actual quality statement on this issue, you would have to have a lot of experience and that comes from checking blood sugar frequently to obtain lots of scenarios and analysis. There truly are so many variables to consider, such as what was eaten earlier, how much exercise was done, and whether there is a possibility of sickness or stress. Making a determination from a brief study or only checking once a day, in my opinion, cannot yield a quality determination. As mentioned at the beginning of the book, the 360 concept—frequent checking—will provide insight for you to make a quality decision and will improve your understanding of blood sugar maintenance. I can say that when extreme blood sugar lows and highs did occur, 95% of the time, we understood why and what mistake we made. It is very rare if you check frequently, document your results and analyze what occurred on a daily basis that you will have a surprise low or high and you do not understand why. You will be thinking, "Oh, wow I forgot to factor in that there was no fat or protein for lunch" or "I forgot about the soda." There will be times, occasionally, when you just want to eat bad high fat and high-sugar foods and this is fine but being aware of what might happen and what you can do to quickly correct a super-high or super-low blood sugar is a key in maintenance. Consider more blood sugar checks if you do not have a continuous monitor. For people without diabetes, keeping fats and proteins in range is key to avoiding extreme hunger/low energy episodes in my opinion.

Adding Exercise—Another Ingredient in the Mix

As explained to me when my daughter was diagnosed upon initial maintenance education, think of fat and protein as six-hour blocks in the chain of your diet. If at any point one of those six-hour blocks has little or no fat (making it weak), that chain could break, meaning your blood sugar drops, and someone without diabetes, you may feel famished. I don't want to overwhelm you but add exercise to the mix and it gets even more complicated because exercise can combat high blood sugar. Why, sometimes, did my daughter have high fat/protein but still, her blood sugar dropped rapidly? Maybe, it was because she was active or exercised that day. A friend of mine who has a teenage daughter who is insulin-dependent and using a pump method told me that exercise does not always have the same effect on her daughter's blood sugar. If she is going to softball practice, she is most likely doing a similar amount of exercise each practice. It might not be the exercise that is causing the fluctuation; it may be that she is eating different amounts of fat and protein before practice. For example, if one day she has a fast-food meal (fries and a burger) before practice and the next day she has a home-cooked meal of spaghetti, the fat, and protein could be affecting the strength of the "safety net." Eating low fat and protein can be very dangerous if you are exercising or being very physically active. Quality fat and protein are the best foods to eat before exercise. However, super-high fat can turn the safety net into a springboard, sending the blood sugar right back up. Finding your perfect meal with fat and protein to act as a safety net before exercise/physical activity can only be achieved by checking and documenting to learn. Exercising after a meal that is higher in fat/protein than you'd normally eat, can help blood sugar stay in range or get back in range. Ask your doctor for your daily recommended fat and protein and recommended amounts before exercise.

Documenting Exercise Is a Bonus!

Documenting the foods that you eat and keeping track of activity also is the only way to best learn the puzzle of blood sugar management. If you have been learning by documenting the foods that you eat and your blood sugar numbers, you will have a 100% chance of making a better game-time decision and avoiding big spikes and drops in blood sugar. You will, especially, be better equipped to decide in a roller coaster situation!

Hats off To You—One of The Hardest Scenarios

A mom or caretaker or someone assisting a middle school or teenager who has diabetes, a healthy appetite and plays sports/dances/cheers. This scenario can be very challenging with the unhealthy high fat and sugar of the American diet, intervals of exercise, adolescent emotions, and growth. This requires some intense management, and I don't believe enough experienced insight to assist is provided or available. If you are having trouble, I understand that it is not easy. In a world where new products, theories, and competitive medical manufacturers dominate, one can become quite confused with what to use and how to manage blood sugar. My advice is to document daily, taking notes of all foods and exercise and how insulin levels are affected. Remember to review the notes and analyze what happened and why. I remember becoming quite robotic in my notes and forgetting to actually review them at the end of the day. Whether you are keeping track in a notebook, your phone notes, or a helpful diabetes App, you will learn from your tracking and analyzing! You may not have to always do this, but you need to learn, and, in my opinion, this is the only way to learn. Doing this consistently for at least a couple of years will enlighten and saturate you with precise knowledge of your situation.

In conclusion, sugar, carbohydrates, fat, protein, and exercise or lack of exercise, sickness, and stress all determine blood sugar and hunger. **To make it easy, the best advice that I can offer after years of caring for my daughter is to try to keep it "consistent" with what you eat and check blood sugar frequently. Here are more tips on how to maintain consistency and level your blood sugar and hunger.**

Good News: Checking frequently or more often to learn for a few years can establish knowledge that will allow you to understand and not have to check as frequently in the future. It is a few years that will educate you and possibly lessen or avoid hypoglycemia (low blood sugar) or hyperglycemia events (high blood sugar). Gaining this initial insight is the foundation of your knowledge for diabetes maintenance—like the fact that you cannot do well in high school and college without a solid grade school education. This initial learning will provide instinctual experience later on.

Consistency Takes Precedence Over All

When my daughter was in high school, I spoke to the school nurse frequently. We spoke about consistency and the importance of it when you have diabetes. She mentioned the swings in blood sugar numbers of the students that were using pump methods to manage their diabetes, a tool that allows you to take insulin, without injecting needles, as and when you need it. You can set the pump to deliver different rates of insulin at different times. This can be convenient because you don't need to take the time to deliver insulin via injection. However, if you don't understand the effect unhealthy high fat and high sugar content in foods can have, and you feel that because you are on the pump and can eat whatever you want, you most likely will still have swings in your blood sugar. A pump product that feeds insulin into your body does not know if you are going to go for a jog after eating or if you are going to take a nap. Some pumps have a feature where you can add your exercise along with your current blood sugar and the amount of carbohydrates you plan on eating and your pump will then use the settings that you have entered to calculate the amount of insulin you need. However, if there is no feature on the pump, it may not be able to calculate accurately. Educators may tell you to be cautious of high fat and protein but if there is no feature on the pump that calculates this factor, it is up to you. The pump does not know if you had fried chicken three hours earlier or if you had a grilled chicken breast. The fried chicken "lingers more intensely" for 6 or more hours and makes it harder for your blood sugar to drop. In other words, you may need more insulin than the pump calculates due to the fried chicken. Skipping a meal may allow the insulin to work quickly and easily bring down your blood sugar, but sometimes it drops too fast, and this can be dangerous. Many insulin-dependent people and caretakers of insulin-dependent people are confused and don't understand why one day everything works and the next day the "roller coaster" effect is happening. The swings may be worse if you are feeling like you can eat whatever you want because now you have a pump and can fix it easily with a press of a button. **The nurse and I agreed that the need for consistency in the diet was still so important.**

When learning about diabetes, how fat and protein are released slowly in your body and the fact that this can affect blood sugar, is not often discussed or taught in detail. Probably because it is complicated (and maybe you want to throw this book out the window!). However, it is an avoidable problem if you just keep your fat and sugar intake consistent and avoid high sugar and high-fat foods. This means reading the fat and protein grams on items that you buy and eat; researching the amount of fat and protein in fast food and restaurant items; and determining a good range for grams of fat and protein in your daily diet. Your doctor, dietitian, nutritionist, or endocrinologist can assist you with determining this for you.

Being On Guard for Too Much Fat/Protein - Examples

Two meals with the same amount of carbohydrates may have a different impact on blood glucose levels because of a prior high-fat (20 g or more) and/or high-protein (25 g or more) meal, which delays digestion and absorption of carbohydrates and may cause some insulin resistance for hours after the meal.

Examples of high-fat and high-protein meals:

- Creamy or cheesy pasta dishes

- Fast food: pizza, burgers, fries, etc.

- Curries and other Asian meals

- Pastries and desserts

- Chocolate

- Chocolate milk

Tips:

1. Check your blood sugar for 2–3 hours (or when your doctor suggests) after eating high-fat or high-protein meals. Make a note of when your blood sugar is high and what foods elevate your blood glucose, so you start to learn and remember.

2. If you are eating a high-fat or high-protein meal, avoid high sugar before and after—have a low-sugar drink or water.

3. For someone without diabetes: Avoid eating high-fat and high-protein meals, but if you do, drink water before, during, and after instead of sugary drinks. Your pancreas is fixing your blood sugar levels now but is working hard to do so when you eat high sugar, high fat, and high protein. Be kind to your pancreas and avoid high sugar and high fat/protein.

Broken Down Further!

Here are some examples of how high fat and sugar interact and affect blood sugar:

These are just examples from my experience of how blood sugar may react. Everyone is different and monitoring your blood sugar and documenting your own results is the best way to learn how your body will react. Someone with insulin-dependent diabetes should always count carbohydrates and adhere to the formula and diabetes maintenance suggestions provided by their doctor. These examples are for awareness.

Breakfast: a pastry (high fat) for breakfast, lunchtime soda, and a sandwich.

Effects on someone who is insulin-dependent:

The high fat from the morning pastry may be released slowly, making it hard for your given insulin to drop your blood sugar. Then a soda with high sugar at lunchtime may spike the already elevated blood sugar and the blood sugar becomes even higher.

Effects on a non-insulin dependent person:

The high fat from the morning pastry is being released slowly, causing your pancreas to work hard to drop your blood sugar. Adding a soda with high sugar at lunchtime may cause your pancreas to work even harder to keep blood sugar in range. You may feel fatigued, tiredness, extreme hunger, and/or jittery

A better choice for breakfast and to have a more consistent day would have been peanut butter, cottage cheese, or egg salad on whole-wheat toast instead of a high-fat pastry. Low-sugar yogurt, oatmeal, fruit, cottage cheese, homemade smoothies with no added sugar or syrup, breakfast wraps, healthy pancakes, and healthy muffins, are all great choices for breakfast.

Lunchtime party: pizza and cake (very high fat and carbs), dinner spaghetti and soda.

Effects on someone who is insulin-dependent:

The high fat and protein from lunch will be released slowly and may keep blood sugar from dropping and the soda with the pasta at dinner may spike the blood sugar even higher. Having a low-sugar drink with spaghetti or water at dinner may help the insulin drop your blood sugar more easily.

Effects on a non-insulin dependent person:

Your pancreas will not have to work as hard to keep your blood sugar at a good level if you have water with the spaghetti at dinner. You may feel fatigued, extremely hungry, and/or jittery throughout the evening if they drink soda at dinner.

A better choice would be to have cake OR pizza for lunch but NOT BOTH. Maybe save the cake and eat it with dinner as dessert and have water to drink. Choose pizza and a side salad or cake and a salad or eat just a few bites of the cake and take the rest home or dispose of it.

Dinner: Creamy Chicken Alfredo and cheesecake for dinner, before bed cereal and orange juice.

Effects on someone who is insulin-dependent:

The high fat and protein from dinner may be released slowly, possibly making their blood sugar higher. The bedtime cereal and the sugar in the orange juice may spike the already elevated blood sugar even higher, resulting in high blood sugar throughout the night.

Effects on a non-insulin dependent person:

Your pancreas will work very hard to keep your blood sugar low all evening and again before bed. You may feel fatigued, extremely hungry, and/or jittery.

A better choice would be to skip dessert when having such a high-fat dinner such as creamy Alfredo and having a low-sugar drink or water instead of orange juice before bed would be a better choice.

One More Extremely Important Tip that Many Do Not Know!

I have seen my daughter's blood sugar "get stuck" in a high range from a previous very high-fat meal like a burger and fries. It would take multiple insulin shots to get her down to a normal blood sugar range. We learned, when this happened, to go slow with corrections with insulin because an avalanche (fast drop in blood sugar) can happen. It is a dangerous game for someone who is insulin-dependent to eat high sugar and high fat and then aggressively try to correct it. For us, if a correction was made with insulin to reduce blood sugar and it did not work, the second time we would try just half of the insulin that is recommended for a second attempt at stabilizing. It might seem as though the first correction may have not worked but it still counts and doing the same correction a second time can be too much. **If you have diabetes and you find yourself on this roller coaster, check your blood sugar more frequently because this scenario is when we experience the most surprises. Talk to your doctor follow his recommendations.**

You Can Improve the Roller Coaster Effect! Here are four ways to avoid the roller coaster effect:

First — In-House Inventory

Becoming consistent with your fat, protein, and sugar begins in the grocery store. Pay attention to the fat, protein, and sugar content of the foods that you frequently eat by looking at the labels. Trying to incorporate some consistency in these numbers is the first step. Try to keep fat content, per serving, in the single digits or close to single digits per serving. Buying drinks and snacks with consistent sugar (no more than 25 grams) can be very helpful. If your favorite iced tea is 28 grams per serving, remember that you can still buy it but add a little water to your glass before filling it with the tea to bring that iced tea sugar content down. If a favorite cookie has 30 grams of sugar, just eat half if you are trying to keep sugars under 15 grams per meal. Pass up high-sugar, fat, and protein items but if you have a true favorite just eat less of it to meet your target amount of fat, protein, or sugar! So, give your kitchen a makeover and get rid of super-high-sugar and high-fat unhealthy products; if they aren't there, you can't eat them! It will be hard at first, but you will remember which foods are not good and you will zoom past them in the grocery store thereafter.

Acknowledge that you will need some WILLPOWER to avoid these foods. Many things are right at our fingertips, but is that always good? Some in our younger generations, in my opinion, are not familiar with saving for years to buy something or having to wait for food or fun. The ability to control desires is fading. Some of us remember our parents and grandparents who smoked cigarettes and would quit by just putting them down and never picking the habit up again. Where did they get the willpower to do this? It can be done! Be strong at work, home, and the grocery store; if you don't buy it, you can't eat it. The more sweets and unhealthy foods that you have lying around in your home, the more you will eat.

Second — Remember portion size!

A food item may only have 8 grams of fat but if you eat 4 times the recommended portion size that is 32 grams of fat. If you overeat this product one day and not the next, your fat intake will be inconsistent, as will your calculations for maintenance even though this product may not be too high in fat. Overindulgence will increase your fat intake as well as your calories. For someone without insulin-dependent diabetes, this will cause inconsistency in your diet, your mood/energy, and possibly your ability to lose weight.

When eating out, be cautious of the portion size and calories in items described as doubles, triple-deckers, stacked, deluxe, XXL, club, large, buckets, platter, premium, thick, stuffed, ultimate, and bowls. Avoiding these larger items will decrease your fat intake. Instead, go for singles, smalls, regulars, original, and small count items.

Third — Dining-Out Choices

If you are a frequent out-to-eat or fast-food junkie, it is going to be a little work because you most likely won't get the nutrition facts for the food you are ordering. You can cut your portion size by choosing a smaller version. If you want to know exactly how much fat is in your selection, there are some great nutritional apps available now that can help you calculate fast food and restaurant food nutritional values. If you are unable to use apps, many restaurants will list the calories of meals on the menu. Compare the meals on the menu to see which have lower calories and choose the lower options because, usually, they are lower in fat as well. Some restaurants even have the calories of drinks listed. Be cautious of what you add to your meal: sides and drinks will add calories, fat, protein, and/or sugar as well.

A good rule to follow is simply to decrease the amount of fat you consume. For example, skip fattening combo meals and fried combinations such as burgers, wings, fries, milkshakes, prime rib, creamy linguine, French toast, and bacon. Many people know that these items are not considered healthy and therefore do not eat them every day but will eat them occasionally—thus creating the sometimes-high-fat, sometimes-not-high-fat scenario (the roller coaster effect). Staying away from unhealthy high fat consistently will help you keep your fat intake more consistent. This is a difficult suggestion, I know, but the less frequently you indulge in these items the more you will be aware of the effects when you do.

Fourth — Follow a Basic Diet Structure

One of the best tools for someone with diabetes or a person who wants to lose weight or maintain a certain weight is to learn about a "basic diet". Learning how much fat, protein, and sugar you should eat with each meal and actually trying to achieve this will help you.

It seems like some of us are just blessed with a twin-turbocharged V8, 1,600 horsepower metabolism, and don't ever need to follow a basic diet. That was definitely me when I was young, and I believe it was like that for both of my parents. However, my family did follow a basic diet daily because that is how it was in the beginning and middle of the last century. When my daughter was diagnosed with diabetes, I was given a paper and told to follow it for success. This was a basic diet plan for a two-year-old. (see pic). This was the first time that I actually saw a basic diet on paper. Although I had done this for years, I was now learning about it. We all hear about basic diets and meal plans but how many of us actually try to use one or stick to one? I am showing you so that you can see the consistency of the meal plan. This is not a diet listing food to buy and eat for breakfast, lunch, and dinner (that would be easy). This is a list of the structure and the amounts of main nutrients you should eat for breakfast, lunch, and dinner. Devising your own meal plan is a good start to becoming consistent. With the help of a nutritionist or doctor or online help, find a plan best designed for you. At first, it may seem too difficult or disciplined but try to follow the basic concept of eating at certain times a day and eating similar amounts of nutrients/meals. If a meal plan is too much for you to follow, just try being consistent to start with. Here are a few ways to start, with baby steps, incorporating some meal plans into your life:

Create your meal plan by first setting times for your three meals, breakfast, lunch, and dinner, around the same time every day, with snacks in between if needed. Make sure your mealtimes fit your schedule. See the meal plan chart. Set a goal to stick with this format. If you have a fluctuating schedule, consider packing food to stay on time. Constant grazing and or random eating is not part of a good meal plan. Small healthy snacks in between are okay.

With the help of a doctor, dietitian, nutritionist, or online calorie calculator, determine your daily caloric intake. Also, determine your starch/carbohydrate (for example, pasta, bread, popcorn, crackers, tortillas, cereals, rice, oatmeal) amount in grams that you should eat per meal/snack. For now, just concentrate on carbohydrates. In the example chart provided for my young daughter the starch/carbohydrates determined were breakfast = 38 g, lunch = 30 g, and dinner = 38 g with snacks being 15 g. These numbers are, of course, very low due to the age of my daughter at the time (19 months old). With the internet, diabetes/dieting has never been easier, just google or use an app to see the carbohydrate content of what you are eating. For example, if I search the internet for "how many carbs does an apple have" it comes up as 25g total carbohydrates. At the time, my daughter may have only eaten half of an apple (12 g) and therefore she would have 26g left to eat. (38 – 12 = 26). A half-cup of instant oatmeal (14g) and a ¾ cup of milk (8g) would amount to 34g. An ounce of Cheddar cheese at 4g would be close to 38g for breakfast with water to drink. She would have achieved her total amount of meal carbs through oatmeal, fruit, milk, and cheese. It is that easy to count your carbs and fit them into your daily chart. If this sounds complicated, stay with me, because it really is not that hard. This incorporates consistency and a quality diet which is very important for your success in achieving a healthy diet.

Determine the carbohydrates you are about to eat, either by looking at the package label, the internet, or a carb-counting book, and fit them into your breakfast, lunch, or dinner whichever it may be. See if it will fit into your suggested numbers for a meal. If not, maybe eat half or three-quarters. Your goal is to fit the number of carbs that you eat into your suggested meal carb count. Average daily carbs could be 225 to 325 grams and if you break that up into 3 meals and 3 snacks it can look like this for a total of 300 daily carbs:

Breakfast: 75 g

Snack: 25 g

Lunch: 75 g

Snack: 25 g

Dinner: 75 g

Snack: 25 g

An average deli sandwich for lunch may have approximately 54 grams of carbs, and you would still have 21 grams of carbs for a drink (75 – 54 = 21). Choosing a pickle that may have just 1 carb is going to be a way better choice than potato chips. We all have our phones on us constantly so it will be pretty easy to determine carbs once you have your customized chart complete.

In our daughter's case, we were advised to include fats and meats (Cheese, peanut butter, eggs, chicken, tuna fish) to prevent blood sugar from dropping too low (the roller coaster effect that I've discussed). Fat and meats are a safety net when consumed in proper amounts and they are healthy, not unhealthy high fat or trans fat. When you search on the internet for the carbs of a food product, for example, you may see that the fat, protein, and calories may also be provided. You can also keep track of these and get an idea of what amounts work best for you.

I was taught that vegetables are very low in carbs and considered free by many, so I was to include them for nutritional value. Vegetables do contain fiber and fiber is great for those who are dieting and for those with diabetes. An article by the Naturelly Family called "10 Amazing Health Benefits of Eating More Fiber" suggests fiber can cut your Type 2 Diabetes risk[4]:

> It's a well-established fact. A recent analysis of 19 studies, for example, found that people who ate the most fiber-more than 26 grams day-lowered their odds of the disease by 18%, compared to those who consumed the least (less than 19 grams daily). The researchers believe that it's fiber's one-two punch of keeping blood sugar levels steady and keeping you at a healthy weight that may help stave off the development of diabetes.

If you do not have diabetes or you have pre-diabetes, this meal structure is still a bonus but if it seems like too much work you can concentrate on just calories. Obtain your recommended calories for a day and divide them as we did for carbs. Every person's daily caloric intake is individual, based on their age, height, weight, gender, and activity plus their personal goals and schedule,

If you need snacks in between meals you may want to divide your day like this:

Breakfast: 475

Snack: 50

Lunch: 475

Snack: 50

Dinner: 900

Snack: 50

Knowing how many calories you should eat for breakfast, lunch, and dinner is a HUGE first step. Looking at what you are eating and knowing how many calories they contain is the next big step and trying to fit them into your daily caloric meal plan is the goal.

Incorporating multiple nutrients into your diet in proper, determined amounts is a bonus to your health. Making sure you have a meal that includes carbs/starch, fat, protein, and vegetables is the ultimate goal. It is not always easy to get vegetables in your diet, but they are super important and big contributors to good health.

If following a basic diet or meal plan seems overwhelming to you, start in "diet kindergarten" by trying a few of these steps and work your way to a bachelor's degree where you can refine your meal plan by learning or being aware of and being cautious of what is in what you are eating. Start slow and understand the concept of eating a well-balanced meal that includes carbohydrates/starch, fat, protein, fruit, and vegetables. As you adjust to having some diet discipline, ease your way into learning about calories, grams of fat, and protein. Stay consistent. Avoid high sugar and unhealthy high fat as much as you can. Incorporating some personal rules/meal plans is a must to achieve your goal. You are allowed and you CAN impose self-discipline and personal "rules" on yourself. Openly discussing your rules when temptation occurs is impressive and can help you and also influence others to follow suit. Reread the chapter on self-esteem if you are struggling.

When my daughter was diagnosed in 2001, we were taught the Exchange Method for managing her diabetes. This method is no longer the primary method taught for diabetes management; however, it worked well for us and still does so I wanted to share what we learned about it.[5]

Here is the chart we received upon diagnosis. This is for a child.

✓ means try

DAILY MEAL PLAN

Meal plan for: _____   Date: 2/12/01
Dietitian: _____   Phone: (___) _____

Breakfast __8:30__ A.M.
2½ Carbohydrate Group (38 g)
  1 Starch _____
  1 Fruit _____
  ½ Milk _____
  0 Meat Group _____
  1 Fat Group _____
  Other _____

Lunch __12:30__
A.M./P.M.
2 Carbohydrate Group (30 g)
  1 Starch _____
  1 Fruit _____
  0 Milk _____
  1 Vegetable ✓ free (NUTRITIONAL)
  1 Meat Group _____
  1 Fat Group _____
  Other _____

Dinner __5:45__ P.M.
2½ Carbohydrate Group (38 g)
  1 Starch _____
  1 Fruit _____
  ½ Milk _____
  ✓ Vegetable (NUTRITIONAL)
  1 Meat Group _____
  1 Fat Group _____
  Other _____

Snack __10:00__ A.M.
1 Carbohydrate Group (15 g)
  1 Starch _____
  0 Fruit _____
  0 Milk _____
  Other _____

Snack __4:00__ P.M.
1 Carbohydrate Group (15 g)
  1 Starch _____
  0 Fruit _____
  0 Milk _____
  0 Meat Group _____
  0 Fat Group _____
  Other _____

Snack __8:30__ P.M.
1 Carbohydrate Group (15 g)
  1 Starch _____
  0 Fruit _____
  0 Milk _____
  1 Meat Group _____
  0 Fat Group _____
  Other _____

NOTE: 1 Carbohydrate Group serving = 15 grams of carbohydrate
Total calories per day: __1300__ to __1400__

Here is a blank chart.

Your Daily Meal Plan Structure

Ask your nutritionist/doctor to help you customize it for you.

Breakfast _____ am	Lunch _____ pm	Dinner _____ pm
Carbohydrate Group (____g) ____ Starch _____ ____ Fruit _____ ____ Milk _____ Meat Group _____ Fat Group _____ Other _____	Carbohydrate Group (____g) ____ Starch _____ ____ Fruit _____ ____ Milk _____ ____ Vegetable _____ Meat Group _____ Fat Group _____ Other _____	Carbohydrate Group (____g) ____ Starch _____ ____ Fruit _____ ____ Milk _____ ____ Vegetable _____ Meat Group _____ Fat Group _____ Other _____
Snack _____ am	**Snack** _____ pm	**Snack** _____ pm
Carbohydrate Group (____g) ____ Starch _____ ____ Fruit _____ ____ Milk _____ Other _____	Carbohydrate Group (____g) ____ Starch _____ ____ Fruit _____ ____ Milk _____ Meat Group _____ Fat Group _____ Other _____	Carbohydrate Group (____g) ____ Starch _____ ____ Fruit _____ ____ Milk _____ Meat Group _____ Fat Group _____ Other _____

Goals:
Total Carbohydrates per day: _____
Total Calories per day: _____
Fat/Protein per meal: _____

Creating A Balanced Meal with Healthy Carbs, Fats, and Proteins

Creating balanced meals will improve your blood sugar maintenance and diet efforts and at the same time provide a safety net to avoid low blood sugar.

• Incorporating protein, carbs, and healthy fats in each meal will help satisfy your hunger and maintain stability in your energy levels. The protein and fat slow down the release of glucose (from the carbohydrates) into the blood stream.

• Choosing healthy fats over unhealthy saturated and trans fats can keep blood sugar levels stable and may help reduce high cholesterol as well.

• As mentioned, when you eat carbs alone, they may be absorbed more quickly into the blood stream and "spike" blood sugars. Eating unbalanced meals can trigger a desire to snack later.

- Skipping meals and overeating at others can lead to unstable peaks and valleys in your blood sugar levels and energy levels. Some may not need snacks in between so that is optional based on need.

- It is quick and convenient to use your hand as a reference to determine portion sizes for your balanced meals. However, keep in mind that individual needs will vary; for instance, men and younger people generally need more food than women, and athletes more than sedentary people.

Here are some examples:

Proteins = 1 palm of the hand or 20- 30 g 3–4 oz (85–115 g) cooked meat/tofu, 2 whole eggs, 1 cup Greek yogurt

Vegetables = 1 fist of hand or 1 cup of non-starchy vegetables

Carbohydrates = 1 handful or 20-30 g 1/2-2/3 cup (100-130 g) cooked grains/legumes, 1 medium fruit

Fats =1 thumb or 7–12 g 1 tbsp (14 g) oils, nuts, seeds, nut butter, cheese

Here are just a few examples of meal combinations with balance:

- Pasta and grilled chicken, tofu, or seafood, vegetable
- Rice and grilled chicken, tofu, or seafood, vegetable
- Roasted or baked potatoes, grilled chicken, tofu, or seafood, vegetable
- Whole grain oats/granola mixed with plain Greek Yogurt, berries/fruit
- Whole grain tortilla, fish, chicken, lettuce/cabbage

Balanced salad as a complete meal:

Salad, shrimp/chicken, shredded cheese, beans or nuts, healthy croutons, or whole-grain toast

Balanced Sandwiches:

Whole-grain bread, lean meat (turkey or chicken breast), lettuce/tomato

Balanced Snacks:

- Two whole-grain crackers topped with one slice (1 ounce) of low-fat cheese, and a few slices of avocado or 2 tablespoons of a simple guacamole spread made of avocado, lime juice, and cilantro.
- Healthy crackers topped with peanut butter and apple slices
- Pita crackers and guacamole or dip
- Fruit/vegetable smoothies with protein: yogurt, kefir, milk, almonds, protein powder, peanut butter, non-fat dry milk

Literature Cited in this Chapter

1. Von Frankenberg AD, Marina A, Song X, Callahan HS, Kratz M, Utzschneider KM. A high-fat, high-saturated fat diet decreases insulin sensitivity without changing intra-abdominal fat in weight-stable overweight and obese adults. *European Journal of Nutrition*. 2015;56(1):431-443. doi:10.1007/s00394-015-1108-6
2. Fetters KA. 10 everyday things that spike blood sugar. EverdayHealth. November 10, 2023. https://www.everydayhealth.com/hs/type-2-diabetes-care/everyday-things-spike-blood-sugar-pictures/?utm_source=twitter&utm_medium=socia
3. WebMD. 20 reasons for blood sugar swings. October 11, 2022. https://www.webmd.com/diabetes/ss/slideshow-blood-sugar-swings
4. Naturelly Family. 10 brilliant health benefits of eating more fibre and how Naturelly Jelly can help. February 11, 2021. https://naturelly.co.uk/10-brilliant-health-benefits-of-eating-more-fiber-and-how-naturelly-jelly-can-help/
5. Gilles G. The exchange method for managing diabetes. March 10, 2023. https://www.verywellhealth.com/exchange-method-managing-diabetes-3289496

CHAPTER 14

Treats in Schools (Parents Don't Skip This Chapter!)

Disclaimer: The next chapter does not cite a specific school or schools. It has been written to make the reader aware of scenarios that are very possible concerning what your child may be exposed to and consuming at school. It is important to remember that as generations move through schools, new parents can change policies and bend rules and vice versa. If you are concerned about your child's weight and or health, I recommend talking to their teachers, other parents, the school nurse if there is one, and definitely your child. Ask your child what they have eaten at school and or after school in any extracurricular activities. If they have a lunch account online, take a look at what they are purchasing to eat. This is how you can find out what is going on at your particular school.

The Way it Used to Be

I attended elementary school in the 1970s and high school in the 1980s. The only place in the school that we ate was in the cafeteria at lunchtime from what I remember. There were rarely any snacks in the classroom. We did not eat in the gym or the auditorium. We either brought a bagged lunch or we purchased a school lunch. The school lunches were served on trays with meat, some kind of starch, a vegetable, and sometimes a bun or a salad. There wasn't a salad bar or any other choices. There wasn't a dessert, snack-candy area, or cart where you could purchase more food after you ate lunch, either. My memories of candy consist of Halloween time and at my brother's baseball games when my mom would let me buy candy at the concession stand.

The Way it is Now

This chapter was the hardest chapter for me to write. Since my daughter was diagnosed with Type 1 diabetes, I had to deal with generous people who loved to provide candy, treats, and snacks for whatever reason, whenever and wherever—and that included school. Why do Americans love to treat children with desserts and candy?

You might be wondering how often this happens, or you may be passing up this chapter because you think that this does not happen regularly in your child's school. **Here is something to think about: if your child does not have diabetes or any allergies, then why would you be notified if they are receiving a treat or snack in school?** Most moms that I've spoken to over the years had no idea that their child was receiving treats in school on a regular basis. Most people throughout my kids' school years, thought that there was a "no treats" policy in the school. There was, well, sort of. If you are a working mom, how often are you at school? Do you go to parties when parents are allowed to come in? I know that every school is different, but when my girls were in elementary school, in a class with 22 to 25 kids, only a handful of moms came to the school events, and they were usually the same moms every time. It is very hard if you are working to attend the school events and parties, so how would you know what was going on at parties? If your kid did not have a food allergy or diabetes, you would not be notified every time a treat was brought in for a birthday recognition, PTA event, or any other random celebration.

Regardless of a no-treat policy, when my kids were in elementary school, there were multiple ways that treats and snacks would make it into the school. I was facing two problems: first, the candy and snacks interfered with diabetes and raised her blood sugar. Second, if the entire class received candy and snacks, and my daughter did not, this would be hard on her psychologically. Some teachers were using the "treat bucket", which was filled with candy and distributed as a reward system for good behavior and/or good grades. Birthday celebrations for the children were another way that treats made it into the school on a weekly basis. Every child had the opportunity to bring in a treat to celebrate their birthday. If the child's birthday was in the summer when school was not in session, they were able to choose a date during the school season when they would like to celebrate their birthday in school.

One year a teacher wanted to get all the summer birthdays out of the way, so she made a special week for the summer birthdays. Every day of that week, someone was providing multiple calorie-busting treats! Then, there was the PTA that would occasionally bring in the treats for the children for different occasions. Most of the time, this was for holidays or for events to raise money for their organizations. At one point, they supplied popsicles after recess just because it was hot. Other random treats that would come in were brought in by a speaker or if the school decided to celebrate something, such as the 100th day of school or to kick off a fundraiser.

Snacks also made their way into the school for state testing. The decision was made to provide a pre-test snack because some kids did not eat breakfast. For the week or 10 days of testing, every child—whether they ate a good breakfast or not—was offered juice and a bag of popcorn or crackers, cheesy crackers, cookie crackers, etc. Again, I am faced with excluding my daughter from the fun of receiving a snack in school while all the other kids participated in the "treat time." I am very fortunate that the school nurse always worked with me and let me know ahead of time what the snack would be for the day. To compromise, I would give my daughter extra insulin to cover the extra snack. We met in the middle, she would have the snack, but not the juice, and she was happy with that.

Middle school was better because the birthday party celebrations were not allowed and that was a big weekly contributor of treats. However, it never ends. You think that the school is not having snacks, but then you learn that a couple of the teachers are having a pizza party at the end of each month for the class if no one has missed a homework assignment. That is not bad, right? It is only once a month. The point is that it is a reward with food and until we stop rewarding with food, we are not going to change the obesity problem.

We do not think we are hurting children with food, but we just might be. The teacher who plans a field trip that consists of a movie with popcorn, candy, and soda, followed by a trip to a buffet restaurant—or any other type of restaurant—for lunch does not think about how many calories this very sedentary field trip may consist of for the children. When people supply treats and snacks for kids, they are trying to be nice and make the kids happy, but in today's world, it has become too abundant. I firmly believe that non-food-related activities like games, exercise, and fitness can make them just as happy. So, why is this not done more often? Well, probably, because it is not as easy as just handing out a snack. If children are participating in exercise or games, then an adult will most likely have to also play or at least supervise. An adult has to come up with an idea and might have to take them to the gym or get permission to take them outside. It is more difficult than handing out goodies.

Other Reasons to Give Kids Treats—The Middle School and High School Cash Cow

You may not be aware that many schools have a post-lunch dessert "snack cart" (usually in middle school and high school) with items such as candy, chips, candy bars, and more. I also heard that sometimes there were French fries on the snack cart as a post-lunch extra. According to a parent on the concession stand committee, these "snack carts" can bring in a whopping $25,000 a year or more for school cafeterias. Do kids need a post-snack after they eat their lunch? No. Does the school cafeteria need an extra $25,000 a year? Of course.

I once told a mom about the "snack cart" and she did not believe me. She called one of her kids into the room and asked them if there was a snack cart after lunch and if they purchased food from it, and the child said yes. The mom asked, "Where do you get the money?" Most schools have the lunch account program where the parents put money into the account every month and the kids use the card or account number to pay for their meal each day, as well as from the snack cart. Unless you look at your child's online account to see what they are purchasing, you may not realize that they are purchasing items other than their lunch.

If your child is in high school, they may be employed and have their own money and can purchase these food "extras" on their own. Worse yet, they may just eat their lunch from the snack cart—junk food for lunch! Having children in school, I have been a volunteer at concession stands and was once on a committee where I learned the wholesale price of "snack food." Most of these items are very inexpensive and can have a huge mark up on them but they still appear affordable. If you put them side by side with a larger size from the supermarket, you may realize that you're not getting much for your money, but when they standalone at a school function and you may be a little hungry, you don't mind paying $2.00 for the tiny item. This is where "snack carts" become gold mines, making them very popular with schools and any organization that needs cash. I have seen these carts try to surface outside of the lunchroom and lunchtime window, to make even more cash at the school and I have complained. However, at the teen stage, kids may not inform a parent about something like this, so you may not know if that is happening. Beware: the rolling snack cart/gold mine can be taken anywhere to bring in big cash at your child's caloric expense.

At the School but not Under School Policy

Some schools have a "no treats" policy, but the after-school clubs and classes do not fall under such a policy. Therefore, if your child is enrolled in an after-school program, such as a reading or math club, Girl or Boy Scouts, Spanish club, etc., they may be getting treats in these environments right before they return home for dinner. Most kids go home after school and like to have a snack before dinner, so this is justified to a certain degree. After-school clubs are usually between the hours of 2 and 5 p.m. The question is, are healthy snacks being served, or are they corn chips, brownies, candy, and so on? As a parent, you may want to investigate because unless your child has diabetes or an allergy, you may not be informed.

Non-School Evening Classes and Sports

My girls attended religious classes for a couple of years, but I withdrew them because of the candy that they were being given. The classes were in the evening, 6 to 7 p.m., and after every class, they would be given candy. I asked why and was told that this is how they keep the class under control. What child needs a bunch of candy right before they eat a bedtime snack? They received chocolate after every voice lesson and an occasional Popsicle after gymnastics. You just never know when someone is going to offer your child sugar. Keep in mind that when you are a have diabetes, you must get your A1C checked every couple of months. Not knowing what and when something is going to be given to your child can add a lot of stress if you are trying to accomplish a good A1C.

The Ripple Effect After a Food Policy Goes into Effect

Several steps can be helpful if you are concerned about your child receiving treats in school. Remember, it may be a continuous and difficult battle, so be prepared. Once a policy has been put into action to stop treats and snacks from coming into the school, many believe that all is good. From my personal experience, I can tell you that it could take a while to end treats in the school and it can resurface in an instant. As one "treat" event is eliminated, a new one emerges. It is a situation where a constant eye is needed to reinforce the policy. Let me give you some examples. After a "no treat" policy was put into effect for holiday and birthday parties, I witnessed candy being brought into the schools being used as bingo chips, and being used to make crafts. This was a way around the policy to get candy to the kids because it was being used for another purpose. I actually heard one mom ask the Homeroom Mom, "I thought we were not allowed to bring candy in?" and the response was, "Well, if it is being used for a game, you can get away with it, everyone is doing it." The school policy stated that any food being brought in had to go through the front desk, then be sent to the nurse so it could be inspected for any food allergens, and then the nurse would notify the teacher. All kids that rode the bus entered through the front door, except the kids that were driven by their parents, who then came in through the drop-off door. The kids started sneaking the treats in through the drop-off door. I actually saw a child carry an entire sheet cake in a large box through that door. It was a way to get snacks and treats into the school without having to go through the front desk and nurse.

Parents or teachers who are new to the school may come up with an idea for treats and not know that a food policy is in effect, or that there are parents who have worked very hard for years to try to minimize the influx of treats because those parents' children have moved onto middle school. With a continuous turnover of parents and students, and sometimes teachers, it is hard to enforce a policy unless it is made a feature of the school. If a school becomes well-known for its beliefs and policies about health and fitness, then less deviation will take place. **This should be a goal of every school.**

The new policy that went into effect during the time that my kids were in school, also tried to limit what was brought in by the PTA representatives, who were steady participants in providing food to the students. The policy had consideration for kids with allergies and basically allowed Popsicles and prepackaged snacks such as pretzels. This eliminated pizza, ice cream, and cupcakes. However, pizza seems to always make its way back into schools, and I am not sure why. I bet if you asked the students if they would rather have pizza at their desks or go outside for an hour, they would choose to go outside. We will not know if we never present the offer. Once America stops using food as a reward, maybe our obesity problem will subside.

What You Can Do

1. Contact the school nurse and tell them that you must know when your child is given a snack. You can tell them that you need to know for allergy reasons, weight concerns, or diabetes concerns. If there is not a school nurse, tell the teacher.

2. Talk to the teacher(s) about non-food related rewards.

3. Let the administration know that you are concerned and ask what their food policies are. Ask if they have a Wellness Committee that you could join or contact. Get their policy in writing.

4. Months before school begins, speak to the administration about placing your child with a teacher who does not use food as a reward.

5. If there are other kids with food allergies, diabetes, or weight concerns, often they are placed together in class. Inquire to see if you can have your child placed in such a class.

6. Let your child know that you are concerned about healthy eating and pack them healthy snacks in their lunch. Who knows? Other kids may follow.

7. If there is a problem with snacks in your child's school, write on the calendar every time your child has a treat or snack in school. At the end of the month, show it to the principal. Sometimes a problem is not noticed or addressed until it is documented on paper.

Documentation is Helpful

The last suggestion, above, is the most interesting. Any time food was being offered in my daughter's class, I was notified because of her having diabetes. Therefore, I always knew when treats and snacks were coming in. I knew that the teachers and the school nurse were aware as well. The nurse and I spoke about the frequency of the treats, and we agreed that it was too much. The teachers knew but did not want to openly comment. Some of them complained about how hard it was to lose weight with the constant influx of treats. One of the traditions of the school birthday parties was that after all the treats were distributed to the students, then the birthday student would get to pick a friend and leave class to deliver leftover treats to all the birthday student's favorite teachers, such as the gym teacher, art teacher, etc. If the teachers did not accept the treat, the birthday child might feel like the teacher did not want to celebrate their birthday. If they took the treat, they had to either eat it or throw it away.

I am pretty disciplined when it comes to staying away from treats. However, if they are handed to me, it's tough to avoid them. I decided to keep track of the days that my child received a treat or snack. Each day, I just wrote on the calendar what the treat was and what the celebration was. At the end of the year, I joined forces with another concerned mom to have a meeting with the school administration. When I presented the calendar, there was disbelief. They said that it seemed unlikely and that they would be questioning the school nurse about it. I never heard anything about it again. My children were soon gone from the elementary level and I did not pursue the issue any longer. It is just like the scenario that I used earlier in this book: one company along the river decides to dump their waste in the river and believes it is harmless but does not realize that 20 other companies are doing the same thing and soon the river is completely polluted. It is very shocking and there can be disbelief when something that isn't monitored surfaces and becomes a surprisingly considerable dilemma. A couple of birthdays a week combined with a holiday party and a fundraiser kick-off can be a very high-caloric week.

Poor Communication

The problem with treats and snacks in schools and after-school activities is that most schools do not have a snack monitor. I do not know if this position even exists in any school. However, there should be a person with that job description. A teacher might want to celebrate one day and give the students a snack, but the teacher does not realize that seven kids in his or her class attend after-school math club, where treats are also given. Maybe one or two of those seven kids also attend an extracurricular activity in the evening, like softball practice or a religious class, and it just so happens that treats are given in those activities as well. Now you have a few kids that received a treat for a classroom celebration at 2 p.m., math club treats at 4 p.m., dinner and dessert with their family at 6 p.m., and a treat at their softball or religious class at 7:30 p.m. This does not even take into account that a kid may have bought something off the post-lunch snack cart. Wow!

How likely is this to happen? Very likely, from what I have learned through my experience; and that is a problem. **None of the adults realize that other adults that day were giving the children treats and even if they did know, would they care?** Here is a calendar I created to show the impact of just the treats given in school to an 8-year-old moderately active child by counting monthly calories and expanding them over a one-year period.

Sunday	Monday	Tuesday	Wednesday	Thursday	Friday	Saturday	Possible Extra Weekly Calories from treats in school
	1	2 4pm Math club candy 240 calories	3	4 1pm Birthday treat cake 350 calories 4pm Math club candy 230 calories	5	6	820 Extra Calories
7	8	9 4pm Math club bag of Pretzels 230 calories	10	11 4pm Math club Gummy s 200 calories	12	13	430 Extra Calories
14	15	16 4pm Math club Potato Chips 300 calories	17	18 4pm Math club cookies 140 calories	19	20	440 Extra Calories
21	22	23 4pm Math club candy 300 calories	24	25 4pm Math club mini frosted donuts (2) 100 calories	26 1pm Birthday treat Cupcake 241 calories	27	641 Extra Calories
28	29	30 Math club packaged crackers 140 calories	31	1 Math club packaged cookies 200 calories	2	3 2pm School celebrates spring with pizza slice 300 calories	640 Extra Calories
							2971 Total Possible Monthly Extra Calories from Treats/Snacks in School.

Using this month's total as an average for possible extra calories given in school, in 9 months (average number of months in a school year) total extra calories from treats/snacks given could be …….. **26,739** Total Yearly.

This calendar is just an example of what could happen in school and after-school classes. It does not calculate what happens at home, after dinner, or during evening activities and the weekends.

If parents knew that their child was already being given treats in school, would they reconsider an evening ice cream trip? Yes. Should a parent be the one who gets to enjoy "treating" their kid? I believe so. Are treats best used to help "control" kids? Rewards are great to help kids learn and encourage them to behave, but not caloric treats that can, over time, harm a child by making them overweight or even obese. Reward them with fitness, games, non-food gifts, stickers, privileges, recognition, etc. If you decide to try to make a difference in your child's school, emphasize these points!

Now let's compare this to a monthly calendar I created that gives healthy snacks:

Calories of Possible HEALTHY Treats/Snacks Given Outside of Lunchtime in School.

Sunday	Monday	Tuesday	Wednesday	Thursday	Friday	Saturday	Possible Extra Weekly Calories from treats in school
	1	2 4pm Math club Box of Raisins 130 calories	3	4 1pm B-day treat Cheese Popcorn 58 calories 4pm Math club Multi-grain crackers 130 calories	5	6	**318 Extra Calories**
7	8	9 4pm Math 100 calorie pack cookies	10	11 4pm Math club Whole wheat crackers 177 Calories	12	13	**277 Extra Calories**
14	15	16 4pm Math club Jell-O 70 calories	17	18 4pm Math club Carrot sticks 50 Calories	19	20	**120 Extra Calories**
21	22	23 4pm Math club Red Delicious Apple 95 Calories	24	25 4pm Math Oatmeal Raisin Cookie 130 calories	26 1pm Birthday treat Freeze Pop 45 Calories	27	**150 Extra Calories**
28	29	30 Math club Clementine 35 calories	31	1 Math club Baked Potato Chips 110	2	3 2pm School celebrates spring Orange & Cheery Ice Pops 40 Calories	**185 Extra Calories**
							910 Total Possible Monthly Extra Calories from Healthy treats in school.

Using this month's total as an average for possible extra calories given in school, in 9 months (average number of months in a school year) total extra calories from **HEALTHY** treats/snacks given could be …….. **8,190 Total Yearly.**

Until parents, school administration, teachers, daycare attendants, and everyone else who is giving your child a treat understands this problem, it will never end. If you decide to try to change the way it is, you will have a big challenge ahead of you.

The Balancing Act – What I learned

A balanced diet is not just about the kind of food that you eat, it is about eating at certain times. Most diet structures allow for snacks in between meals, but they do not recommend cupcakes, ice cream, pizza, or candy for these snacks. Between-meal snacking should consist of healthy choices, such as crackers, cheese, fruit, vegetables, yogurt, nuts, etc. because of their low glycemic quality. This basically means that they are kind to your pancreas. Your pancreas works hard to keep your blood sugar low on a daily basis. When you eat foods high in sugar and unhealthy fat, your pancreas has to work even harder. Eating meals and snacks too close together can spike blood sugar because your blood sugar from your previous meal is not stable or low enough yet or your pancreas is still working hard at keeping your blood sugar low. Eating more carbs/sugar too soon after a meal can be too much. Timing is a key factor in a balanced diet.

This is a fact I learned from doing the 360 Test: you need time between meals to let your pancreas work and recover from a meal. Eating too close together or eating too big a snack between meals is a guarantee to spike blood sugar or make your pancreas run a marathon, even if you do not have diabetes. It can also cause indigestion. After a meal, give your pancreas a couple of hours to do its job. One of the most difficult tasks about diabetes is to stay on a schedule and eat meals when you are supposed to. Factors such as sports, events, celebrations, church, travel, etc., can make it difficult to eat a meal when you are supposed to eat. I am speaking about this based on first-hand knowledge.

Taking on the Challenge

My best advice is to talk to the teachers and try to get them to join the "fitness craze" with you. Rewarding students with fitness should be the theme for every school in the United States. I actually was very fortunate to have a school that heard my cries for help. Many of the teachers were on board and wanted to change the reward options. I saw huge progress during the last year of my youngest daughter's elementary schooling. Traditionally, upon 4th-grade graduation, there had always been a graduation ceremony that was similar to that of a senior, where a cap and gown were worn and the students received a diploma on stage and then went to the cafeteria after for cake, pizza, and soda. The event was a very sedentary event with a high caloric intake. However, my youngest daughter's last year in elementary school was celebrated with a softball competition. It was held at a local park with two softball fields, tennis courts, and a jungle gym, and a competitive bounce house was brought in. The classes were divided into nine teams and as four teams played on the two fields, the other teams were able to run freely doing any of the activities of their choice. The bounce house was very popular, identified by the long line to participate; the jungle gym was booming and many enjoyed tennis. A disc jockey was brought in and karaoke was an ongoing event that was very popular and fun to watch. Volunteers also participated; they took turns playing limbo with the kids. I was a chaperone and watched the children have so much fun! The kids were all told to bring a water bottle, and they had to bring their own lunch. The only food that was provided was snow cones.

All it takes is a shift in thinking and a little imagination. Our brains are molded to think that celebration and reward equal food, and that needs to change. Kids love anything that breaks up the normal day, but it doesn't have to be a cupcake.

Reward with Fitness or Non-Food Items/Ideas

Elementary School

1. Game time, story time, movie or video time
2. Game time, story time, and movie time in a "special place"
3. Dollar store items: pencils, pens, markers, erasers, bookmarks, books, rulers, magnets Frisbees, paper, activity game sheets
4. Arts and crafts
5. Be the helper, teach the class, sit by friends, eat lunch with the teacher, eat lunch outdoors, have lunch with your BF (best friend) in the classroom
6. Dance to your favorite music in the classroom
7. Show and tell
8. Field trips or sports competitions
9. Computer time, phone time
10. Gym day—play in the gym
11. Extra recess, extra anything listed above

12. A banking system—stickers or money or a form of money to save for privileges
13. Listen to music while working
14. Talk Time at the end of class

Middle School

1. Reduced homework or no homework
2. Dollar store items: pens, pencils, stickers, erasers, bookmarks, books
3. Listen to music while working
4. Art or talk time at the end of class
5. Extra credit, recess, talk time, music, art time, phone time, computer time
6. Movies or videos
7. Assemblies
8. Field trips or sports competitions
9. Eat lunch or have class outside
10. Coupons or gift cards

High School

1. Reduced homework or no homework
2. Listen to music while working
3. Art or talk time at the end of class
4. Eat lunch or have class outside
5. Extra credit, recess, talk time, music, art time, phone time, computer time
6. Movies or videos
7. Assemblies
8. Field trips or sports competitions
9. Coupons or gift cards
10. Drawing or writing contests for donated prizes
11. Allow students to read aloud poetry or stories that they have written

The activity could incorporate fitness; for example, in math, count the number of hops for one person to hop across the playground and multiply it by the number of kids in the math class to get the total number of hops. For celebrations, such as the 100th day of school, students could have a 100 fitness challenge: 100 jumping jacks, 100 jump ropes, 100 steps, etc. Watching documentaries or movies that have won awards will teach about quality writing. Have a discussion after.

In CCD or Sunday school classes, which often take place in the evening before bedtime, if the class is cooperative for the last ten minutes, they can have a cool-down where they get to stand and stretch, do twists, touch toes, listen to music, or watch a movie. The Bible is full of adventures: they could be allowed to stand and emulate or act out the actions of someone in the story as the story is told or played.

The above list of non-food rewards can also apply to after-school dance classes, sports, or cheerleading practices.

Proof

In May 2015, I interviewed a high school student to get an opinion about the early process of mis-educating kids about food in the education system. Here is what was said:

> As a high school student, I can attest that being rewarded with food still happens, even at my age of 17. For students in most of the advanced classes at my school, every Friday is a treat day to reward us for the work we have completed throughout the week. As an incentive to attend after-school tutoring sessions, teachers stockpile large amounts of food for us to eat while learning outside of the classroom.
>
> Outside of extracurricular snacking, another issue is the quality and cost of the lunch that is provided. To purchase a deli sandwich, a side salad, and pretzels would cost a student upward of $6. But to buy a fried chicken sandwich and fries, it only costs $3 or $4. $3 a day times 180 days in a school year really does add up, which causes the chicken and fries to always win out. Unfortunately, the fried chicken sandwich and fries are much larger portions, which keep us full, but leave us to feel lethargic and, for lack of a better term, "blah" after we eat them. But because it is bigger and cheaper, it is almost as if we have no choice. The worst part about it is that my school is one of the top in the state when it comes to food-choice quality. We win awards for our lunches when, at their very best, they are subpar.
>
> Chances are that your child's school is worse. Many people have turned to pack lunches due to the greater variety of choices and the lesser price, which is good but shouldn't be necessary. The school should provide proper nutrition. In other countries

similar to the United States, they do. Children are taught at an early age the value of good nutrition. Lunches in France, Germany, Sweden, Brazil, and almost any other country you can imagine, have fruits, vegetables, and rice, and proper portion sizes. A typical elementary school lunch in the U.S. consists of popcorn chicken, mashed potatoes, and a cookie. The peas and fruit cups are only there because of state requirements and 99% of the time they look so unappetizing that children are almost forced to throw them away.

Meanwhile, in France, lunch consists of steak, FRESH fruit, green beans, carrots, and a slice of cheese. In South Korea, it is rice, fish soup, and fresh vegetables. For more examples, all you must do is google "school lunches throughout the world" to see the difference. If you think there is no way your child would eat this, you might be right, but that is only because they have grown up on the standard American diet of junk food. Maybe if they weren't fed a diet that primarily consisted of a potato cooked in various ways from their first day of school—if not before—they would be open to eating these healthier lunches. In the first place, these international lunches are so nicely prepared that they look better than any school-made lunch I have ever seen. They even look better than most American homemade meals. The U.S. needs to instill proper nutrition information into their children from a young age, just as the rest of the world does, or the obesity epidemic will reach epic proportions.

CHAPTER 15

Balance Food and Activity – A Must Know!

Balancing food and activity is a very important part of a healthy diet! You just have to pay attention and be aware. This will probably be the easiest tip you will read in this book. Small changes over time can be very rewarding!

Energy is another word for "calories." Your energy balance is the balance of calories consumed through eating and drinking compared to calories burned through physical activity. What you consume through eating and drinking is ENERGY IN. What you burn through physical activity is ENERGY OUT. You burn a certain number of calories just by breathing air and digesting food. You also burn a certain number of calories (Energy Out) through your daily routine. For example, children burn calories just being students—walking to their lockers, carrying books, etc.—and adults burn calories walking to their car or into work, going shopping, etc. An important part of maintaining energy balance is the amount of Energy Out (physical activity) that you do. People who are more **physically active** burn more calories than those who are not as physically active.

The same amount of Energy In (calories consumed) as Energy Out (calories burned) over time = weight stays the same

More Energy In (calories) than Energy Out over time = weight gain.

More Energy Out than Energy In (calories) over time = weight loss.

Your Energy In and Energy Out don't have to balance every single day. It's having a balance over time that will help you stay at a healthy weight for the long term.

It is a good idea to find your Estimated Calorie Requirement as mentioned earlier to get a sense of how many calories (Energy In) you need on a daily basis. It is best to find estimates that include your activity level or (Energy Out) so that you have a balance of food and activity.

Here are some Energy Out examples that you may see on an Estimated Calorie Chart that includes activity:

A. Sedentary means a lifestyle that includes only the light physical activity associated with typical day-to-day life.

B. Moderately active means a lifestyle that includes physical activity equivalent to walking about 1.5 to 3 miles per day at 3 to 4 miles per hour, in addition to the light physical activity associated with typical day-to-day life.

C. Active means a lifestyle that includes physical activity equivalent to walking more than 3 miles per day at 3 to 4 miles per hour, in addition to the light physical activity associated with typical day-to-day life.

A good chart will include calorie ranges to accommodate the needs of different ages within the group, gender, and possibly bone structure.

Practicing Energy Balance

Eating just 150 calories more a day than you burn (Energy Out) can lead to an **extra 5 pounds** over **6 months.** That's a **gain of 10 pounds a year.** If you don't want this weight gain to happen, or you want to lose the extra weight, you can either reduce your Energy In or increase your Energy Out. Doing both is ideal for achieving and maintaining a healthy body weight.

Some Ways to Cut 150 Calories (Energy In)

- Drink water instead of a soda
- Order a small serving of French fries instead of a medium or order a salad with dressing on the side and only use half
- Eat an egg-white omelet (with three eggs), instead of whole eggs
- Put chips in a bowl instead of eating out of the bag and overeating
- Skip dessert

Some Ways to Burn 150 Calories (Energy Out), in Just 30 Minutes (for a 150 lb. Person)

- Take the steps instead of the elevator
- Walk two miles
- Do yard work (gardening, raking leaves, etc.)
- Go for a bike ride
- Dance with your family or friends
- Do yoga before bed

Make your own list of ways that you can reduce calories slightly every day. Make a list of more ways that you can burn extra calories daily and post the lists where you can constantly see them.

Slimming Down for Festivities

If you know that you are going to a party and there will be a lot of irresistible food and beverages, eating fewer calories for a few days prior can help to reduce your post-party weight gain. You can relax a bit at the party when it comes to food, as you will have positioned yourself for a slight gain in your weight. Or, you can increase your physical activity level for the few days before or after the party, so that you can burn off the extra energy. This is practicing energy balance.

The same applies to your kids. If they'll be going to a celebration and eating cake and ice cream—or other foods high in fat and added sugar—help them balance their calories the day before and/or after and encourage them to be physically active after a celebration with an abundance of treats/sweets.

CHAPTER 16

The Easiest Step – Pack Your Lunch

The Way it Used to Be

In Chapter 7 "Fast Food", you learned that fast food and snacks were not as readily available 40 years ago as they are now. Gas stations, also known as service stations, were much different and you definitely did not purchase a meal or any hot food there. Candy, chewing gum and drinks were about the most that you could purchase at a service station. Ballparks and sporting venues were not about food; they were more about the event—your reason for being there. I went to see a ton of rock concerts and quite a few sporting events, and don't remember eating during the event. When my family went to the amusement park, my mom and dad packed our food, brought a cooler that we carried into the park and left on a picnic table until it was lunchtime. But this isn't a popular idea now because of all the available fast food.

What You Can Do

I had a conversation with a friend who is unhappy with her weight. She has an office job (very sedentary), is older, and no matter how much she works out, she still finds herself gaining weight. After a few months of a personal trainer and still no improvement, I asked her what she eats for lunch. I knew that she did not eat breakfast; therefore, I assumed that she was usually starving by noon every day. She told me that she eats fast food. I asked her why she did not pack a lunch. She explained that it was impossible to pack a lunch because she did not want to carry a lunch box on the bus; the microwave at her workplace was too dirty; and there was no room in the refrigerator to put any food. I tried for half an hour to convince her that to see the results she wanted, she had to try to make packing her lunch possible. Having a daughter with diabetes, a peanut allergy, and a shellfish allergy makes me the queen of lunch packing. I also, occasionally, pack a healthy lunch for my husband, to assist with saving money. I told my friend about all the different-sized ice packs that are available and that will keep food chilled for four or five hours. I told her to look in her grocery store and online for all the small containers that are available for packing and storing food. I even advised her of some foods that are great for putting in a packed lunch, such as mandarin oranges, peanut butter and jelly sandwiches, raisins, pistachios, salsa and nachos, cheese sticks, yogurt, cereal bars, etc. For those who do not like the drab appearance of a lunch box, there are fashionable insulated containers with matching thermoses. I didn't think that she was listening to a word I said. However, about a month later, she did let me know that she had started packing her lunch occasionally. She said that while it is boring compared to going out to get fast food, she has most certainly noticed a drop in her weight. It seems that eating is almost entertainment or a well-needed, exciting break in the day that we look forward to. If you can break free from that concept a few times a week and settle for just a "not as exciting" meal at your desk or in the office lunchroom, then you could lower your weight, and maybe your cholesterol, all while keeping your wallet fat. It is a mind-over-matter situation; resist the temptation—you can do it!

I have found that my oldest daughter has never minded packing her lunch. It was helpful with her having diabetes because I knew how many carbs she was eating. In elementary school, the cafeteria would sometimes give prizes out to the kids who purchased lunches. My daughter would come home a little sad because she did not get a prize. So, to counter that, occasionally I would put my own little prizes in her lunch box. I would pick up a few things at the dollar store or would write her a note or a joke.

Once in Westchester County, New York, I had the pleasure of working for a Fixed Base Operator (a place where private planes land and take off). One of my jobs was to deliver catering to the planes before they took off and retrieve catering after planes landed. The planes that I was taking care of were owned by some of the wealthiest people in the United States. The nearby catering company that we used was sensational, not just when it came to taste (we often received unused catering), but with their presentation as well. The food at times looked like expensive gift-wrapped items. Occasionally, I would wrap a ribbon around a Tupperware container in my daughter's lunch, put fancy tissue paper around a candy bar, or use pastel-colored cupcake papers to put crackers in. I packed her sandwiches, stews, baked or breaded chicken, tacos, risotto, soups, and many more delicious meals. Over the years, I have had several moms approach me and tell me that their kids wanted lunches just like hers. Most of the time, it was just leftovers from dinner the night before.

A couple of years ago, I went to a professional baseball game with my parents. An older woman was sitting next to my Dad and had brought her own sandwich. She was talking about the venue and how to save money because the food there can be very pricey. If our family is going on a trip, maybe a ski trip, and we have to drive three or four hours to get there, I pack a cooler for two reasons: First, because I don't want to stop and take the time out to get fast food and, second, to save money because that's money that we can use in a quality restaurant for a more nutritious meal when we get to where we are going. The kind of meal where I can sit down and relax and have a server bring it to me. I don't want to eat a meal I pay for in my car. So, at any point in our journey when someone is hungry, they can reach in the car and grab a ham sandwich or peanut butter and jelly sandwich. I also usually pack some potato chips or pickles and something to drink; I find that is enough to hold us until we get there. I've also packed sandwiches for long dance competitions, field trips, and amusement parks. If you pack a lunch once a week, you may save $12 and if you multiply that by 52 weeks, that is $624 that you have saved. If you pack twice a week, you may save $1,248.

As for calories, a fast-food meal can be up to 1,200 calories and a packed lunch may be a mere 600; just think about the calories you can cut. In a year of packing your lunch, twice a week, you could cut 62,400 calories from your diet! Would you be curious to see if that would affect your weight? Try it! Sandwiches are easy to pack. I like wrapping them in waxed paper and taping them shut, kind of like how you might receive a deli sandwich. Small Ziplock bags are great for potato chips or pretzels and mini-Tupperware containers can hold pickles or carrots.

Packing salads is also an option but may require a little more work. Soups and stews can also be packed. At work, you can reheat them in the microwave. If a microwave is not available, there are thermal food containers that keep your food hot/warm. Once you get the hang of it, it does not become so time-consuming and the financial and weight loss benefits are great.

There are many healthy snacks and packaged options available now. Combining these with a healthy sandwich, salad, or soup/stew can be a good idea.

CHAPTER 17

Learn to Flip It—The Most Important Tip in This Book

The information and opinions in this chapter can change and vary among experts and should be read for awareness purposes only. A nutritionist or doctor can help you customize your intake to match your personal dietary needs.

Many people purchase processed and packaged food and are so trusting they never think to look at the label on the back to see what they are eating. I strongly suggest taking a peak. I believe it would help prevent weight gain, diabetes, and disease if you become familiar with what you are consuming and learn to consume healthy food.

Here Are Some Tips

Serving size

First, check out the serving size and if there is more than one serving per container, that means that you should be pouring "a serving size" into a cup, plate, or bowl and only eating that much. It also means that the nutritional information listed is just for ONE serving size and if you eat double the serving size, you must double the amounts of fat, calories, carbohydrates, etc. If you eat triple the serving size, then you must triple the amount, and so on. If you are interested in eating proper portions, learning to read labels is a must! Let's say a serving size for a packaged snack is ¼ cup and you eat ½ cup, then you have to double the fat, the calories, and the sodium. If it is a ¼ cup and you eat 1 cup, then you must quadruple the information. Serving sizes are there for a reason. What is considered the proper serving size is different in many parts of the world. Be sure to flip your package over and check to see the recommended amount you should eat and FOLLOW IT.

Servings per container

Servings per container would most likely be for prepackaged food. Let's say you have a box of cookies. If the box says 100 calories in a single serving and 5 servings per container and you eat the whole box, then you have consumed 500 calories. Eat the serving size, but not the whole box!

Calories

Calories, simply put, are your source of energy. Every single food has calories, some more than others. The recommended caloric intake for the average person who does little to moderate physical activity is 2,000 calories to maintain their weight. However, if you are someone who eats closer to 3,000 calories a day, scaling back to a 2,000-calorie diet could help with some weight loss. It probably is best to see your doctors and have them recommend a target daily calorie goal for you.

No matter if you want to maintain or lose weight, reading the label is one of the most important things you must do. If you are about to consume a 500-calorie dessert, ask yourself if that slice of cake, that bowl of ice cream, or that huge, sweet coffee is worth a quarter, or more, of what you are recommended to eat in an entire day. And, as always, remember to adjust the information according to the serving size you choose. Yes, the back of your ice-cream carton says that you are only eating 140 calories, but that's for a quarter cup. When was the last time you ate just a quarter cup of ice cream? Chances are you are consuming close to 600 calories by the time you eat the whole bowl. Again, serving sizes are very important and are meant to be followed to help you stick to your recommended caloric intake.

A general guideline for calories is that 40 calories in a single serving is low, 100 is moderate and 400 plus is high.

Recommendations

The U.S. Institute of Medicine recommends that Americans consume about 20–35% of their total calories from fat. Every gram of fat contains nine calories. This means a person who eats 2,000 calories a day should consume fewer than 78 grams of fat per day.

Calories from fat versus calories from carbohydrates

People who are trying to maintain or lose weight should focus on the total calories and fat consumed, rather than on whether the calories come from fat, carbohydrates, or protein. "It's pretty clear that the source of the calories is really not important," said Walter Willett, chairman of the department of nutrition at Harvard School of Public Health, in a July 2008 *Time* magazine article.[1]

Total calories versus calories from fat

When looking at the percentage of calories that come from fat, it is important to consider the total calories per serving. Food that gets 60% of its calories from fat—a large amount—may not be unhealthy if the total number of calories per serving is low. For instance, food that has 60 calories per serving but gets 60 percent of its calories from fat, has only 4 grams of fat per serving. Good foods like nuts have most of their calories from fat, but they give you sustained energy and will help keep you feeling full longer. Calories from fat are not as important to note as total calories, overall, but for higher-calorie foods, they are a good thing to note and keep track of.

Sugar

How much sugar is in this item? I prefer less than 21 grams of sugar and over 25g is getting too high. In my personal experience with monitoring my daughter's blood sugar, when you consume items with a sugar content of 30 or 40g, blood sugar can easily skyrocket.

In my opinion and through my experience, I found natural sugar to raise blood sugar less than added sugars. It seemed to me that natural sugars are not only less aggressive with raising blood sugar, but they are more consistent as well making it easier to calculate insulin over time. Added sugar can be very inconsistent with how it affects (raises) blood sugar. Added sugar can be a real guessing game and can produce big spikes in blood sugar and this may be due to package labels being incorrect about the measurement of ingredients. I personally found natural sugar to be more consistent.

You may see that an orange has the same amount of sugar as a packaged pastry, but the orange will provide you with energy while the packaged pastry will supply you with weight gain. The American Heart Association says that the maximum amount of sugar a man should eat a day is 37.5 grams and for a woman, 25 grams. To put that in perspective, a single can of soda could have more sugar than a person should eat in an entire day. If you are overweight or obese, added sugars should have no place in your diet. Try to cut them out as much as possible, so that you can focus on being a healthier you.

There are many ways to minimize your added sugar intake. A great one is to take out soda from your diet and drink water. If you can't stand the taste of water, go for unsweetened iced tea once in a while. Be sure to know the alternative names for sugar. There are many, and they include sucrose, high fructose corn syrup (HFCS), dehydrated cane juice, fructose, glucose, dextrose, syrup, cane sugar, raw sugar, corn syrup, and more. If one of these words is in the first three ingredients of something you are about to eat, or if two different types of sugars are in one product, avoid it and find something with a healthier nutritional value. Ingredients are placed in order of the quantity in the product. When any type of sugar is in the first three ingredients, that means it is loaded with sugar. If you are craving sugar, eat fresh fruit. They are sweet and are loaded with natural sugars that are healthy for you. Avoid fruit packaged in syrup. More often, than not, it contains added sugar. Also, be careful when it comes to "low-fat" foods! A lot of the time, to compensate for the lack of fat, these foods are loaded with sugar to make up for the taste. As always, flip the package and read to make sure you know what you are putting into your body! Most people do not realize that they can quench a sugar craving with something small such as a handful of raisins, or a piece of dark chocolate. You don't need 500 grams of sugar to satisfy that craving!

Fat

How much fat is in the product? My personal rule is that the fat content should be in single digits - under 10 g per serving! I make exceptions for cheese, meat, and occasionally, chocolate, but I do not eat these items in excess. I found this works well in controlling diabetes especially if you are consistent. Stay away from the unhealthy bad fats that can eat up your daily recommended fats in one meal.

Fat is an essential nutrient that we need for healthy skin, hair, and nails. It is also an important source of energy. However, consuming too many grams of fat can lead to obesity and put you at risk for heart disease, among other things. When you eat fat, make sure that you are consuming the right kinds of fat. Unsaturated fats are the best to eat. They come from things like fish oil, extra virgin olive oil, avocados, hummus, and nuts. Saturated fats come from animal-based products like dairy and meats. The Dietary Guidelines for Americans encourage you to only consume up to 10% of your calories from these foods.

While saturated fats do cause obesity and heart disease, good fats are very important to put into your daily diet, according to www.helpguide.org.[2] Don't go for that fat-free option all the time. In the last century, when waistlines were slimmer, fat-free options didn't exist! Take this example provided by www.helpguide.org and remember that sometimes fat-free products can have a lot more sugar to make it taste better:

> A walk down the grocery aisle will confirm our obsession with low-fat foods. We're bombarded with supposedly guilt-free options: baked potato chips, fat-free ice cream, low-fat candies, cookies, and cakes. But while our low-fat options have exploded, so have obesity rates. Clearly, low-fat foods and diets haven't delivered on their trim, healthy promises.

Despite what you may have been told, fat isn't always the bad guy in the waistline wars. Unhealthy bad fats, such as trans fats, as well as too much sugar, are guilty of the unhealthy things all fats have been blamed for—weight gain, clogged arteries, and so forth. But good fats such as monounsaturated and polyunsaturated fats, including omega-3s, are healthy. In fact, healthy fats play a huge role in helping you manage your moods, stay on top of your mental game, fight fatigue, and even control your weight.

Myths and Facts About Fats

Myth: All fats are equal—and equally bad for you.

Fact: Trans fats are bad for you because they increase your risk for heart disease. However, monounsaturated fats and polyunsaturated fats can be good for you because they lower cholesterol and reduce your risk of heart disease.

Myth: Lowering the amount of fat you eat is what matters the most.

Fact: The mix of fats that you eat, rather than the total amount in your diet, is what matters most when it comes to your cholesterol and health. The key is to eat more good fats and less bad fats.

Myth: Fat-free means healthy.

Fact: A "fat-free" label doesn't mean you can eat all you want without consequences for your waistline. Many fat-free foods are high in sugar and calories.

Myth: Eating a low-fat diet is the key to weight loss.

Fact: The obesity rates for Americans have doubled in the last 20 years, coinciding with the low-fat revolution. Cutting calories is the key to weight loss, and since fats are filling, they can help curb overeating.

Myth: All body fat is the same.

Fact: Where you carry your fat matters. The health risks are greater if you tend to carry your weight around your abdomen, as opposed to your hips and thighs. Plenty of belly fat is stored deep below the skin surrounding the abdominal organs and liver and is closely linked to insulin resistance and diabetes.

Polyunsaturated Fat and Monounsaturated Fat

These are known as good fats, as most unsaturated fats are, as stated in this article by the Mayo Clinic.[3] The types of potentially helpful dietary fat are mostly unsaturated:

Monounsaturated fat. This is a type of fat found in a variety of foods and oils. Studies show that eating foods rich in monounsaturated fats (MUFAs) improves blood cholesterol levels, which can decrease your risk of heart disease. Research also shows that MUFAs may benefit insulin levels and blood sugar control, which can be especially helpful if you have type 2 diabetes.

Polyunsaturated fat. This is a type of fat found mostly in plant-based foods and oils. Evidence shows that eating foods rich in polyunsaturated fats (PUFAs) improves blood cholesterol levels, which can decrease your risk of heart disease. PUFAs may also help decrease the risk of type 2 diabetes.

Omega-3 fatty acids. One type of polyunsaturated fat is made up of mainly omega-3 fatty acids and may be beneficial to your heart, especially. Omega-3, found in some types of fatty fish, appears to decrease the risk of coronary artery disease. It may also protect against irregular heartbeats and help lower blood pressure levels. There are plant sources of omega-3 fatty acids. However, the body doesn't convert it and uses it as well as omega-3 from fish.

Foods made up mostly of monounsaturated and polyunsaturated fats are liquid at room temperature, such as olive oil, safflower oil, peanut oil, and corn oil. Fish high in omega-3 fatty acids include salmon, tuna, trout, mackerel, sardines, and herring. Plant sources of omega-3 fatty acids include flaxseed (ground) and nuts and other seeds (walnuts, butternuts and chia seeds). Incorporate these into your diet!

Protein

Protein is very important, as it helps with muscle and plays a key role in our body's functions; however, the Dietary Guidelines state that we need only .37 grams per pound of body weight per day for the average sedentary human. If you are 160 lbs., you only need 59.2 grams of protein. In one 12 oz. steak, there are 77 grams of protein. Of course, you need more if you are planning on building muscle, but for the average human, a normal American-size portion serving of steak is more than enough protein for the entire day. If you are a vegetarian there are also plenty of ways to get protein through various beans, vegetables, and grains such as quinoa. Eating protein for weight loss is tricky. My experience has shown that if you double the amount of protein recommended and exercise a lot, then your metabolism speeds up and weight loss is easier. For the same 160 lb. person, 120 grams of protein would be recommended per day. Be careful with your protein intake. Eat enough to support your muscles and activity level but do not go overboard. For someone with diabetes, protein plays a very important role in balancing blood sugar.

Carbohydrates

How many carbohydrates are in the product? A decently healthy snack usually has fewer than 30 grams of carbohydrates per serving size.

While all nutrition needs depend on your weight and activity level, carbs need to be the most personalized. The number of carbs that you eat—while still losing weight—can be nearly double what your best friend or coworker eats, and vice versa. Carbs on a food label can be found under sodium and before protein. Be sure to look at the percent daily value of carbs one serving snack has. While everyone's healthy carb intake is different, the percentage is still a good guideline to go by. One cup of cereal generally has 30–40 grams of carbs which is around 10–15% of your ideal daily intake. Everyone knows carbs come from bread and pasta, but the best source of carbs is actually in the fruits and vegetables that keep you feeling full longer. If you are going to get carbs from wheat sources, make sure that it is whole wheat. White bread, pasta, etc. are much lower in fiber and will therefore make you feel hungry not long after you eat.

Sodium (salt)

Salt makes you retain water and makes you thirsty. If you aren't drinking water, you will be taking in calories from sugary drinks to quench your thirst. Try to keep your salt intake to a minimum to be a healthier you. According to www.Heart.org, the best salt intake is less than 1,500 mg a day. Not all our sodium intake comes from the saltshaker. Most of it comes from processed foods. In fact, only 12% of the salt we eat occurs naturally, and the other 88% comes from unhealthy processed foods. As with all nutrition, if you just limit your intake of packaged, frozen, or processed foods your diet would be so much better.

Percent Daily Value

The percent daily value, or PDV, is self-explanatory. It appears most often on the right side of the nutrition label and tells you the percentage of the daily value for each nutrient (usually it is all the fats, cholesterol, sodium, carbohydrates, and protein) in a serving of the food, and reflects the proportion of this nutrient as part of a standard 2000 calories per day diet. For example, a particular bag of trail mix, for a 1/4 cup serving, has 9 grams of fat, or 14% of the DV. But again, the odds of only eating a 1/4 cup, if I don't watch my portions, are small and so, if I eat a half cup, or double the serving size there, it will be 28%. If you are getting more than 25% of any nutrient from one serving of any product, that is a red flag, and you should not consume it.

Fiber

Fiber comes in two forms: soluble and insoluble. Soluble fiber slows digestion and helps control blood glucose and cholesterol levels. Insoluble fiber helps with stool softening. Fiber is very important, as it helps you keep feeling full longer, but only 3% of Americans are getting their daily recommendation.[4] Consuming foods high in fiber will reduce the temptation of eating foods that are not as good for you. The average woman should consume 25 grams of fiber a day and the average man should consume 38. To put that into perspective, 38 grams of fiber is the same amount that is in 15 pieces of whole-wheat bread. But there are plenty of other places to get your fill of fiber without the grain overload. Beans and lentils are the best places to find your fiber, but most fruits and vegetables are full of them as well. Healthy cereals generally have around 10 grams of fiber, so you can start your morning off right by getting one of the most important nutrients in your body, plus it will keep you fuller than a non-fiber breakfast!

Fiber is usually found under the carbohydrate section on the nutrition facts label so be sure to flip the package and look for snacks that have at least 4 grams of fiber to get your recommended amount for the day. I usually consider the other information as well, just to see the quality of the snack.

Vitamins and Minerals

To see how many vitamins are in your products, look at the nutrition facts. All the vitamins your product has are listed with their percent daily value. It is good to eat products with a lot of vitamins because it means that they have good nutritional value. The most important vitamins are vitamins A, B, C, D, calcium and iron. It is very important that you get your daily amount of these for a healthy functioning body. Noticing vitamins in a product is a good habit to start because it will encourage you to purchase quality products.

Vitamin A, vitamin C, calcium, iron, and other vitamins are healthy ingredients that I look for in a product. If a product contains NO VITAMINS, then I will most likely not buy it or I will eat it only once in a while.

Chemicals

Does the product have chemicals? America is a very "trusting" nation, but maybe we shouldn't be. By this, I mean that we believe everything that is said to us by our governmental health organizations, even when it may not be true in the long run. Don't you want to know what you are putting into your body? Take a package of regular corn tortilla chips and compare the ingredients to tortilla chips that have sprinkled flavoring all over them. Plain tortilla chips have only a handful of ingredients whereas flavored chips contain things like artificial colors (yellow 6, yellow 5, red 40, sodium benzoate, potassium benzoate, and butylated hydroxyanisole [BHA]). Why would you want to put all those chemicals into your body? Be selective with what you eat! Generally for snacks, if there is a paragraph of ingredients, it is not going into my body! Quick snacks from convenience stores and vending machines can be packed with calories, chemicals, and not much nutrition. Finding your daily caloric intake goal, which should be discussed with your physician, and then "flipping the food" item over to read the calories will be an eye-opener and is a must-learn for healthy eating and proper portion consumption.

Now that you have an education on how to read a product label, it is time to update your cabinets! Go through and select better-quality foods!

Note: Some snack companies have started putting product information on the front of the package. I think this is a great idea.

Literature Cited in this Chapter

1. Ending the War on Fat. TIME. June 12, 2014. https://time.com/magazine/us/2863200/june-23rd-2014-vol-183-no-24-u-s/

2. Robinson L, Segal J, Segal R. Choosing healthy fats. HelpGuide.org. March 13, 2024. https://www.helpguide.org/articles/healthy-eating/choosing-healthy-fats.htm

3. Dietary Fat: Know Which to Choose. Mayo Clinic. February 15, 2023. https://www.mayoclinic.org/healthy-lifestyle/nutrition-and-healthy-eating/in-depth/fat/art-20045550

4. Clemens R, Kranz S, Mobley AR, et al. Filling America's fiber intake gap: summary of a roundtable to probe realistic solutions with a focus on grain-based foods. *The Journal of Nutrition*. 2012;142(7):1390S-1401S. doi:10.3945/jn.112.160176

Chapter 18

Why Try to Prevent Obesity—What You May Not Know

Good Reasons to Get Fit and to Stay Fit

It is important to talk to your kids about healthy eating—and not give up. I started talking to my girls about healthy eating, sugary and fattening foods, and watching their weight before they were 10. Trying to teach them how to eat healthy was quite a battle and one that I feared I was going to lose. It seemed that the constant desire for sweets would never end. Around age 15, I noticed a slight weight gain in one of my daughters. She mentioned that her jeans were tight. A few days later, she informed me that she had put herself on a diet. I told her that she didn't have to go crazy but maybe just cut out some sweets. I told her that I was happy that she was interested in staying fit and concerned about the extra weight that she had gained. Around age 15 or 16 a female is usually done growing and should try to remain the same size for a while.

About six months after our conversation, I noticed that items in our "treat" cabinet were not being consumed. This was really a milestone for me. All my relentless nagging and harping about overeating and consuming sweets too often had finally sunk in. Then a bomb dropped. It was Halloween and I bought Halloween cupcakes like all moms love to do. I showed them to my daughter, and she said, "Mom! I'm trying to diet and I need healthy foods!" This was truly an epic day for me, seeing my kids catch onto a healthy lifestyle. I believe it was the subtle doses of early education about food, and reminders along the way, combined with her own observation of her body. Plus, a few of her fitness friends who worked out at the gym may have inspired her—probably more than I did. I told her that sweets are fine once in a while as a treat or dessert but not several times a day or all day long. **Kids may not realize that sweets used to be a dessert after dinner!** In our society today, sweets are accepted anytime and anywhere. Many very sugary treats today are disguised as "coffee" or a "smoothie" and may not be counted as a treat but should be.

Kids also may not realize that you shouldn't have to keep buying bigger sizes of clothing into your late teen years. When I was young, we did not get new clothes often and if your jeans did not fit, you had to suffer or lose weight. In today's world, some kids receive clothing more often so it may be easy to assume that if an item does not fit... just go and buy something new. I had jeans for at least 5 years after I graduated from high school, and they fit. Let your kids know that when they are done growing in height, they should start watching their weight and help them figure out their goal weight for their height. You can show them and explain the growth chart that suggests a proper weight for your height. You can get one online or from your physician. Change is often so slow that it goes unnoticed until it is very visible. Addressing the issue before things get out of control is always wise in any aspect of life.

Also, leggings were not a popular article of clothing to wear out when I was young. They are considered normal daily wear now inside the house and outside. This easily allows weight gain with no pain. Kids need to be visually aware of their bodies, not because of appearance but as a monitoring method to keep fit for health reasons. Tell them that they will lead a healthier life with fewer complications if they stay fit from the start. Explain that diabetes and many other complications can result from being overweight.

This chapter was very tough for me to write because nobody wants to hear about or talk about these things. However, it is important to know ahead of time what you are getting yourself into if you choose the road of being overweight. Somewhere along the line from the 80s fitness era until now (over 40 years later) the criticism of the issue of trying to look like models and famous people overshadowed and smoke screened a very important goal of staying fit for health reasons. With heartbreaking diseases like bulimia and anorexia occurring, who could argue with the dismissal of caring about what you look like? Striving to stay fit was getting confused with the symptoms of these diseases. I feel that it's important to know that there is a difference between trying to stay fit and starving yourself to look like a famous slim celebrity. The goal should be to stay healthy and fit to avoid problems that result from carrying too much extra weight. No, we do not have to look like a runway model, but we do not have to gravitate to the opposite end of the spectrum either by allowing ourselves to gain 50 to 100 extra pounds, all in the name of being happy with who we are.

A Sneaky Avalanche

So, what exactly is so bad about being overweight? Through media and doctors, one might hear of heart problems and/or diabetes, but that can seem so far off in the future that it may be easy for young people to disregard and not worry about them. However, gaining weight with "no concern or care" can become an avalanche. It starts as 10 pounds of excess weight, then the next year it is 20 pounds, and then 30 and then 40, and the next thing that you know you are 100 pounds overweight at age 60. Ten extra pounds may not be bad but 20 may make it hard to do certain exercises and may hinder your energy level during exercise, which makes working out more difficult. If a task becomes difficult, it is easier to not want to do it.

This is the very beginning of a reduction in mobility. Carrying an extra 20 pounds can lessen your desire to work out or exercise due to the difficulty of the task. When you lack the desire to be fit as well as the desire to exercise, you are setting yourself up for an avalanche of weight gain. A slow consistent gain over a period of 10 or 20 years can leave you quite surprised when you suddenly realize how bad it has become. Here are a couple of comparisons: financial problems; unpaid taxes; drug and alcohol problems; a deteriorating home; a field that hasn't been cut and now is very overgrown. These are all problems that could have been avoided but were not addressed early on and now are much more difficult to fix. Once these problems are out of control, they are harder to correct. The avalanche of gaining weight is the same.

It is hard to stop and get back to where you were when you were fit. Your awareness of weight gain and monitoring your weight at an early age is vital to staying fit. As I mentioned, most of us have heard about the side effects of being obese. If you are obese you are predisposed to heart attacks due to coronary heart disease, heart failure and stroke, high blood pressure, high cholesterol, and diabetes. However, if you are still ignoring the slow avalanche of weight gain and you are thinking of throwing this book out the window right now, here are some uncomfortable and annoying consequences and realities that you may not have heard about and may experience as an obese person:

Bone/Arthritic Problems

Think about carrying 20 pounds of extra weight around each day.

> Every pound of weight gained puts an extra four pounds of pressure on each of your knee joints. So, if you gained just five pounds, it would be like adding 20 pounds to each knee.[2]

Imagine if you put on a vest that had huge pockets in it, and you could put weights in it to "test out" being overweight, we may then understand what life will be like while supporting extra weight. The human body was not meant to continuously support excess weight. Not just knees but feet, hips, ankles, shoulders, and backs all suffer when doing so. Extra weight can put pressure on connecting tissues around joints such as tendons that connect muscles to the bones. Extra pressure on joints can cause the tendons to become inflamed, resulting in tendinitis. It is a long period of carrying excess weight that eventually produces problems for joints, bones, and muscles. Extra pounds can eventually lead to arthritic problems. Once a person reaches a certain level of obesity, because of these problems they can become completely immobile, perhaps needing a wheelchair or they avoid moving at all because of the pain they feel when walking. Being obese can cause swelling in the lower extremities from the pressure of the weight. This can result in chronic changes to the legs and feet. **At this point, exercise will most likely be impossible.** A person in this position has probably not been able to exercise for many years or even decades.

Skin Problems

Skin can only stretch so far! Stretching skin can cause unattractive stretch marks. When skin is stretched too far it can become scaly and open to drain fluid. Infection can set in at this point. In some cases, it can be difficult for healing to take place due to the excess fat surrounding the infection because fat does not heal very well.

Infections

Air/oxygen heals infections. A bandage is used when a wound is open and needs protection or when it's bleeding. Once a wound begins to heal the bandage should come off and the fresh air will aid in the healing process. When a person is very obese certain areas may be covered by excess skin and cannot receive proper air, light, and or oxygen. For this reason, being overweight can lead to increased skin infections or other infections.

Depending on your body stature, when carrying an extra 50 plus pounds you may develop a pannus or "apron" (skin hanging over the skin). A pannus can capture moisture. With daily movement, rubbing under the pannus can occur. A yeast infection can develop from trapped moisture, continuous rubbing, and lack of air. A short person may have an increased chance of developing this, as a tall person will have more area for their weight to be distributed, so less "hanging." The genital area and under the arms are other areas that may not receive much air when carrying excessive weight and may be more susceptible to infection. In extreme cases, these "fungal" excoriations (untreated cellulitis infection of the skin) can become chronic, needing a wound VAC to treat them. They may require special incisions and/or retention sutures.

Pickwickian Syndrome and Sleep Apnea

I remember after eating a delicious home-cooked meal, my grandfather, as he was standing to leave the table, would rub his belly and smile. This was a kind gesture to let everyone know that he enjoyed the meal and it was a huge compliment to my grandmother for her exceptional cooking. I remember being in my early thirties when a dozen of my male friends lined up at a pool party for a side shot photo of all of their rather large stomachs. A large stomach can be a sign of wealth (living well) and/or enjoying life, but what is the downside? Pickwickian Syndrome can be a huge downside. This is when you are uncomfortable lying flat on your back because your stomach is putting too much pressure on your diaphragm and lungs, making it hard for you to breathe. People with Pickwickian Syndrome can get help by using a CPAP or BiPAP (positive air pressure assistance) to help them with breathing. Without assistance, OSA (obstructive sleep apnea) can occur, and that is when you stop breathing during sleep. This can cause daytime fatigue or sleepiness and poor attention, and problems at work can result. Eventually, OSA can lead to heart or lung problems. It can also result in anxiety and depression. A lack of sleep can have many other negative effects on the human body.

Visceral Obesity

Excess intra-abdominal adipose tissue accumulation is often termed visceral obesity. This fat is a build-up wreaking havoc on your insides by putting pressure on your organs, bones, and muscles. That is right, fat does not just grow outward. Visceral (inner fat) can actually smother your organs as it expands both ways.

Hygiene—Hard to Reach

I am just going to touch lightly on this as no one really wants to read about such issues. Yes, when drastically overweight, it may become hard to reach certain areas and take care of daily hygiene needs. Also, due to increased fat, trapped moisture can cause bacteria to thrive. Therefore, an increase in E. Coli infections, yeast infections, and urinary tract infections can result. Especially for women. Obviously, these conditions can result in decreased sexual desire as well as other problems.

Surgery Complications and Wound Compromise

Obese patients' wound healing compared to patients of normal weight is substantially different. There is strong evidence indicating the association between obesity and problematic surgical outcomes. This is especially true in relation to wound healing, such as increased wound infections, wound separation, wound failure, and fascial dehiscence as well as general surgical complications. Excess fat can make it harder for a surgeon to find and reach the bone or organ, so the surgery can be more difficult and possibly take longer. A longer or larger cut in the skin may be the result, thus making wound healing longer and more difficult.

Chronic Pain Syndrome

As your weight increases, you are more likely to have chronic pain syndrome or long-term pain. In obese persons, general and specific musculoskeletal pain is common and weight loss for obese pain patients appears to be an important aspect of overall pain rehabilitation according to the *Journal of Pain Research*.[3]

Other Thoughts to Consider About Obesity

There are other consequences of being morbidly obese that you might not have considered. Many nursing homes do not accept patients that are 350 pounds or more. When you are morbidly obese, you may require special chairs and/or beds, and a special hydraulic lift may be necessary to lift you from a bed if you become incapacitated. You may be required to purchase two seats on an airline. At a morbidly obese weight, you may not be able to function or have any type of mobility in your senior years.

If morbidly obese, you could be denied a CT scan if your body size is too large for the scanner. A CT scan can be a very important test before a surgical procedure or for determining your state of health.

These situations illustrate why it is important to know what your normal weight range should be. It is based on your height and gender. Again, you can meet with your doctor and/or review an "ideal weight chart" online to find it. If you are in range, strive to stay in range and check often to continue this path. If you are not in range, then set goals to try and get in range. If you are out of range, don't panic, just make daily changes and over time you will see results!

Literature Cited in this Chapter

1. Kelly FB. What weight means for your bones. OAC. Fall 2013. https://www.obesityaction.org/resources/what-your-weight-means-for-your-bones/

2. Okifuji A, Hare BD. The association between chronic pain and obesity. *Journal of Pain Research*. Published online July 1, 2015:399. doi:10.2147/jpr.s55598

CHAPTER 19

Why Aren't You Exercising? Exercise and Physical Activity

We spoke about balancing energy in and energy out. To achieve this, exercise or physical activity is needed. For some, the word exercise is taboo, like the word "scale." Professionals in the medical and dietary industries sometimes tiptoe around the subject of exercise and use less harsh descriptions such as physical activity or just activity. The "E" word is too much to bear. There can be some confusion though as to what exactly physical activity and exercise are. According to my mom, she always got plenty of exercise daily as she went up and down the steps in her split-level home.

Both exercise and physical activity have benefits

Both are beneficial to your health and, on a regular basis, they are one of the most important things you can do for your health. Routine exercise and physical activity can help with not only balancing energy in and energy out but also much more. They:

- Strengthen your bones and muscles
- Improve your quality of life
- Control your weight
- Reduce your risk of cardiovascular disease
- Reduce your risk for Type 2 diabetes and metabolic syndrome
- Reduce your risk of some Cancers
- Improve your mental health and mood

- Improve your ability to do daily activities and prevent falls, especially for older adults
- Increase your chances of living longer

The more that you do, the more you increase these benefits.

Finding Your Fitness Level

Your doctor may have told you to start exercising or incorporate some physical activity into your daily routine. You may be wondering whether it will make a difference or whether you can do it. Finding your beneficial fitness level depends on your desire, your doctor's recommendations, and your physical capability. Most importantly, no matter what your current fitness level is, activity and moving are going to be a benefit. If you have a chronic health condition, talk with your doctor to find out if your condition limits, in any way, your ability to exercise and/or be physically active. Work with your doctor to come up with a plan that matches your abilities.

Exercise and physical activity are different

Exercise is a form of physical activity that is planned, structured, and done to improve at least one aspect of your physical fitness, for example, strength, flexibility, or aerobic endurance. Exercise will have more of an impact on improving the bulleted list above.

Physical activity includes any body movement that contracts your muscles to burn more calories than your body would normally do at rest or while in a sedentary state. Everyday physical activities such as performing housework, walking, or taking a hike keep your body moving and count toward the recommended amount of weekly physical activity and will contribute toward improving the above list of benefits.

Trying to incorporate exercise or physical activity into your daily or weekly routine is a little tougher in today's busy world and the excuses are plentiful:

Falling Into the Luxury of an Excuse?

There are the **burst exercisers** who are the people who never exercise but then once a year decide to try and get in shape. They buy exercise equipment or join a gym and it lasts only briefly and ends abruptly.

There is the **nostalgic group** who tell you all about how much they used to exercise when you ask them if they are currently exercising.

There is the **futuristic group** who are going to join the gym when or after some event takes place: "As soon as I...", "When I get back from...", after the New Year, etc.

There is the **medical condition** group who absolutely cannot exercise due to an injury, a condition, their medicine, and/or doctor's orders.

The **hangover group**! If you are hungover on your workout day, you just might not work out.

The **pop-up group**. Something always pops up and takes priority over your mentally scheduled workout plans.

Personally, I think I am in the "**can't accelerate group**," where you are committed to exercising once a week and do not miss it, but desperately want to exercise more than once a week. Most of us want to be committed exercisers who commit to a daily or multiple times-a-week workout. Which group are you in?

What's important is that you avoid being sedentary and inactive. Even 60 minutes a week of moderate-intensity aerobic activity is good for you. Toss out the excuses!

What Research Studies Have Found

Reduce Your Risk of Cardiovascular Disease

If you get at least 150 minutes of exercise each week, you can reduce your risk of heart disease and stroke. For example, moderate-intensity aerobic activity can put you at a lower risk for these diseases. Regular exercise might also help you to reduce your blood pressure and improve your cholesterol levels.

Reduce your risk of Type 2 Diabetes and Metabolic Syndrome

Regular physical activity can reduce your risk of developing Type 2 diabetes and metabolic syndrome. Metabolic syndrome is a condition in which you have some combination of too much fat around the waist, high blood pressure, low HDL cholesterol, high triglycerides, or high blood sugar. Research shows that lower rates of these conditions are seen with 150 minutes (2 and a half hours) a week of at least moderate-intensity aerobic activity. And the more you do, the lower your risk will be. If you already have Type 2 diabetes, regular physical activity can help control your blood glucose levels.

Reduce Your Risk of Some Cancers

Being physically active lowers your risk for many types of cancers. For example, research shows that:

Physically active people have a lower risk of colon cancer than people who are not active.

Physically active women have a lower risk of breast cancer than people who are not active.

Reduce your risk of endometrial and lung cancer. Although other factors may also be involved, some findings suggest that your risk of endometrial cancer and lung cancer may be lower if you get regular physical activity compared to people who are not active.

Loss of bone density comes with age so it is important to protect your bones, joints, and muscles from early on in life. Not only do they support your body and help you move, but keeping bones, joints, and muscles healthy can help ensure that you're able to do your daily activities and be physically active. Research shows that doing aerobics or muscle-strengthening and bone-strengthening physical activity of at least a moderately intense level can slow the loss of bone density that comes with age. Muscle-strengthening activities can help you increase or maintain your muscle mass and strength. Slowly increasing the amount of weight and number of repetitions you do will give you even more benefits, no matter your age.

A hip fracture is a serious health condition that can have life-changing negative effects, especially if you're an older adult. However, research shows that people who do 120 to 300 minutes of at least moderate-intensity aerobic activity each week have a lower risk of hip fracture.

Regular physical activity helps with arthritis and other conditions affecting the joints. If you have arthritis, you might consider 150 minutes (2 hours and 30 minutes) of moderate-intensity aerobic activity, like cycling at less than 10 miles per hour, or 75 minutes (1 hour and 15 minutes) of vigorous-intensity aerobic activity, like cycling at 10 mph or faster, each week. Another option is to do a combination of both. A rule of thumb is that 1 minute of vigorous-intensity activity is about the same as 2 minutes of moderate-intensity activity.[1]

Improve Your Mental Health and Mood

Once you establish a regular exercise routine, you will most likely notice the good feeling that you get after finishing a workout. Some people become exercise "junkies," needing this good mental feeling regularly. Exercise can help keep your thinking, learning, and judgment skills sharp as you age. It can also reduce your risk of depression and may help you sleep better. Research has shown that doing aerobics or a mix of aerobic and muscle-strengthening activities 3 to 5 times a week for 30 to 60 minutes can give you these mental health benefits. Some scientific evidence has also shown that even lower levels of physical activity can be beneficial.[2]

Improve Your Ability to do Daily Activities and Prevent Falls

A functional limitation is a loss of the ability to do everyday activities such as climbing stairs, grocery shopping, or playing with your grandchildren. If you're a physically active middle-aged or older adult, you have a lower risk of functional limitations than people who are inactive or sedentary. If you already have trouble doing some of your everyday activities, gradually starting aerobic and muscle-strengthening activities can help improve your ability to do these types of tasks. Research shows that doing **balance** and **muscle-strengthening activities** each week along with **moderate-intensity aerobic activity**, like brisk walking, can help reduce your risk of falling.[3,4]

Need More Convincing to Exercise?

The Mayo Clinic confirms exercise helps boost your mood and 7 more benefits and advice[5]:

Seven benefits of regular physical activity

Exercise controls weight

When you engage in physical activity you burn calories and consistency is the key.

Exercise improves mood

If you need an emotional lift or need to blow off some steam after a stressful day, a workout at the gym or a brisk 30-minute walk can help. Physical activity stimulates various brain chemicals that may leave you feeling happier and more relaxed. You may also feel better about your appearance and yourself when you exercise regularly, which can boost your confidence and improve your self-esteem. (Many people become addicted to the good feeling you experience after working out).

Exercise boosts energy

Winded by grocery shopping or household chores? Regular physical activity can improve your muscle strength and boost your endurance. Exercise and physical activity deliver oxygen and nutrients to your tissues and help your cardiovascular system work more efficiently. And when your heart and lungs work more efficiently, you have more energy to go about your daily chores.

Exercise promotes better sleep

Struggling to fall asleep or to stay asleep? Regular physical activity can help you fall asleep faster and deepen your sleep. Just don't exercise too close to bedtime, or you may be too energized to fall asleep.

Exercise puts the spark back into your sex life

Do you feel too tired or too out of shape to enjoy physical intimacy? Regular physical activity can leave you feeling energized and looking better, which may have a positive effect on your sex life. But there's more to it than that. Regular physical activity can lead to enhanced arousal for women. Men who exercise regularly are less likely to have problems with erectile dysfunction than men who don't exercise.

Exercise can be fun

Exercise and physical activity can be enjoyable. It gives you a chance to unwind, enjoy the outdoors, or simply engage in activities that make you happy. Physical activity can also help you connect with family or friends in a fun social setting. So, take a dance class, hit the hiking trails, or join a soccer team. Find a physical activity you enjoy, and just do it. If you get bored, try something new.

The bottom line on exercise

The health benefits of physical activity far outweigh the risks of leading a lethargic, sedentary life. Exercise and physical activity are a great way to feel better, gain health benefits, and have fun. As a general goal, aim for at least 30 minutes of physical activity every day. If you want to lose weight or meet specific fitness goals, you may need to exercise more. Remember to check with your doctor before starting a new exercise program, especially if you haven't exercised for a long time, or have chronic health problems.

If you are no longer in school or college, read the next chapter, "Post-Organized Sports," to learn why you might be having trouble getting into an exercise routine!

Literature Cited in this Chapter

1. Physical Activity for Arthritis. United States Centers for Disease Control and Prevention. January 5, 2022. https://www.cdc.gov/arthritis/basics/physical-activity/index.html

2. Pearce M, Garcia L, Abbas A, et al. Association between physical activity and risk of depression. *JAMA Psychiatry*. 2022;79(6):550. doi:10.1001/jamapsychiatry.2022.0609

3. Thomas E, Battaglia G, Patti A, et al. Physical activity programs for balance and fall prevention in elderly. *Medicine*. 2019;98(27):e16218. doi:10.1097/md.0000000000016218

4. What You Can Do to Prevent Falls. United States Centers for Disease Control and Prevention. 2017. https://www.cdc.gov/steadi/pdf/STEADI-Brochure-WhatYouCanDo-508.pdf

5. Exercise: 7 Benefits of Regular Physical Activity. Mayo Clinic. August 26, 2023. https://www.mayoclinic.org/healthy-lifestyle/fitness/in-depth/exercise/art-20048389

Chapter 20

Post-Organized Sports

Active in School—Not Active After School

The life you lead after participating in high-school or college athletics can be a time when some people lose touch with exercise and fitness because they are unable to take charge and coordinate their personal workout routines. It's not hard to understand how this might happen. In high school and college, organized sports have a coach(s) AND other teammates who are relying on you to be there. Your parents and friends are coming to see you play and you don't want to disappoint them. Also, acquiring a scholarship may have played a big part in your dedication, but then it all ends when school is over. There is no one and nothing counting on your dedication. Some people seek out and sign up for non-school sports/leagues that are organized by companies, fraternities, alumni, or just individuals who have come together. But it can be hard to find these post-school organizations and you may not feel as comfortable because you may not know as many people on the team as you did in school and those commitment factors aren't there. For those who cannot find a team of some sort, you may be faced with trying to organize your own fitness routine. This can be challenging.

Arranging Your Post-Organized-Sports Fitness Life

Although moderate physical activity such as brisk walking is safe for most people, most health experts advise that you talk with your doctor before you start an exercise program if you have heart disease, diabetes, or a current injury. It is good to know what type of exercise you want to engage in before talking to your doctor. Here are some ways to figure out what type of exercise you might enjoy and will stay dedicated to.

First, you have to decide what time of day would be best for you to exercise and how much **time** you can dedicate to fitness each week. Are you a morning person? There are morning boot camps and sunrise exercise classes, and most gyms are open very early or even 24 hours. Determining a good "time" can help you be faithful.

Second, are you a self-disciplined person or do you need outside help? Are you into doing activities **solo, with a friend, or in groups**?

Third, you will also consider how much **money** you would like to invest into your fitness routine. There is a saying, pay for fitness now or pay for medical expenses later. I don't know if that is true, but it is my decision to give the former a try rather than the latter. If you are considering a gym, less expensive memberships may be at the YMCA. Many gyms offer discounts or specials throughout the year. An average-priced gym would be one where you receive or choose no individualized attention from a personal trainer. You decide what you do every day instead of someone instructing you. The most expensive gyms are those that incorporate a personal trainer and dietary counseling.

Lastly, you will have to choose a **fitness category.** If you aren't sure, possibly mimic what you enjoyed in school. Look back at the training you did while you participated in sports, whether it be basketball, football, gymnastics, dance, swimming, baseball, or any other athletic team. Was there a particular stretching, core, upper and lower body, or cardio sequence that you really enjoyed and would like to recreate to the best of your ability? Think about what part of that school activity you really enjoyed. Choosing a fitness category that you enjoyed in the past can help prolong your current dedication. You may not be able to keep the same pace or lift the same amount as you did in your younger years, but chances are you can still do the basics. After you have an idea about these questions, you can start planning your post-school fitness routine.

Here are some examples to help you determine a post-organized-sports routine to fit the kind of person you might be:

Completely Independent Person

1. Gym membership or home gym

2. Workout videos

3. Solo sports: jogging/running, swimming, bicycling, inline skating, bodybuilding, weightlifting, surfing, skiing, snowboarding, skateboarding, rollerblading, kayaking, gymnastics, yoga, dancing, trampoline, diving, paddle surfing, bowling, badminton, cross-fit, triathlon, ice skating, motocross, equine sports, surfing, boxing, judo, pole dancing, figure skating

4. Fitness apps: There are some fantastic fitness apps for someone with self-motivation.

Please see the chapter *What To Look for In a Workout App* for suggestions on how to find a fitness app that is best for you.

Independent Person Who Needs a Little Structure

Fitness Instruction:

These people are always doing some form of exercise or fitness, but they are just not 100% dedicated or consistent. They know that all it would take is a signature to become more consistent (i.e. signing a contract to join a gym or fitness organization)! There are tons of classes that men and women can sign up for that can help you stay in shape, including spin classes, yoga, hot yoga, boot camps, muscle pump, aerobic step classes, and more. Look for these classes at your local gyms/fitness centers, schools, and fire halls, and, if you are fortunate, your workplace may have a fitness center or classes. Some of the most recognized classes like Zumba, spinning, Pilates, and CrossFit are long-lasting favorites. New trends in fitness are constantly emerging, such as pole workouts. It is all about choosing what may keep your interest. You may want to sign up for Zumba if you like fun times—the original dance-fitness party is an easy, fun way to get into shape. CrossFit is for those who are serious about getting into shape and gaining muscle, and who are not afraid of in-your-face atmospheres. Whatever type of fitness class you choose, there is something about signing up and paying for six months or a year of instruction that helps you stay committed. Especially if you go a few times and get to know a few people who will greet you when you return and if you miss a class they will ask where you were. Having a set day that is YOUR day or evening to go to your class and work out can help you stay faithful. Taking classes is easy to incorporate into your schedule and can actually mimic the organization you experienced in school. Set your own "practice" schedule as if you were in school. Pick days to attend the classes and stick with it, keeping in mind you must go just like you had to go to school.

Being a coach/fitness instructor:

Helping others can help you stay committed and in shape. Sign up! Commit! Determine how much time you can dedicate to being a coach. Volunteering or a paid position as a coach can keep you in great shape if you join in on the workouts. Once you sign up, you have made a commitment and must stick to it. This is very similar to signing up for sports in high school and college and fits the independent fitness person who needs a commitment. There is a need for fitness instruction help in many areas: personal trainers, yoga instructors, group exercise instructors, assisted stretch professionals, water aerobics instructors, senior living fitness instructors, elementary, middle school, and high school coaches, corporate group fitness instructors, etc. Depending on how much training you want to do to become a coach or trainer will determine who you can help and where you can work. For example, it may take less time and fewer requirements to become certified as a fitness instructor for seniors or as a coach for elementary sports than it would to be a personal trainer at a weight-training gym. I was a cheer coach for three years when my youngest daughter was in middle school. It kept me very busy and in shape with all the practices and cheers/dance routines to learn. Once my daughter was in high school, the coach had to have more requirements and training. I didn't know this ahead of time or I may have planned ahead and received certification. Look online for fitness instruction help and see what might interest you and what certifications you may need and could acquire.

Dependent Person (you need to be dragged out of bed)

These are people who feel as if they need motivation from external sources to accomplish their fitness routine. They may struggle to stick with a fitness routine and/or go long periods (years/decades) without fitness. Here are some important steps and options that can help:

Delete The Mental Block:

I have a friend who is overweight. I asked him if he wanted to review a short science-fiction story that I wrote. He reviewed it as soon as I gave it to him. He loved it, offered a few ideas, and also listed some grammar and mechanical errors for me to fix. I then asked if he wanted to review THIS book. He took it from me but never read it, saying that he just was not interested in the topic. I guess I need to write a sci-fi book about diet and diabetes! Delete the mental block that you might have about why you can't lose weight, get into shape, exercise, and be dedicated. You can do anything if you try!

Ask For Help:

Get the family involved or ask a friend to help you. Let someone know that you want to make a change and need help. Find someone to exercise with you.

Transportation buddy. Take turns driving so that you are responsible for getting someone else there. The pressure of not letting your buddy down can keep you motivated to keep attending practice/classes.

For the dependent fitness person, the most ideal option would be to hire a **personal trainer** who would have a scheduled appointment with you each week and walk you through your workout. However, this can be expensive. Another option might be to return to the type of organization you had in high school or college by signing up for a class but signing up with a friend who is going to stick with it and encourage you to go. Or you can speak to the class instructor and ask them if you can get reminders (emails, texts, or a phone call before class). Tell them that you need help. Sign up for a team or league and ask for encouragement from other teammates.

Signing long-term contracts or commitments can be helpful to keep you going. Attending scheduled classes at the gym by purchasing a *year's worth ahead of time* can save you money and also provide pressure to keep you going **BUT** on top of that, you need a support buddy or someone to remind you to go. I have a friend who purchased a yearlong gym membership once and did not use it! It happens, so you need a partner as well—someone to push you. If you ask the gym owner to reach out and send reminders, they may be willing to help or suggest a workout buddy who travels with you.

Why Do You Need a Workout Buddy?

In 2015 nearly 55 million Americans were members of a fitness center. However, 60% of those never used their memberships.[1] If you cannot find a workout buddy or you don't want to take a chance on spending money on a membership and possibly not going, try to develop a routine at home first. Doing a little at home on a consistent basis for a long time will better prepare you to become a gym junkie. Start with one day a week then increase to two. Mark it on the calendar. Build your habit slowly and stay the course. Your body gets addicted easily and believe it or not, it can get addicted to exercise. Unlike most addictions, this is a good addition.

Getting Back Into the Habit

It is a huge change for someone who has not been exercising for over a decade to jump back into it. So, if you want to test the waters before hiring a personal trainer, signing a year membership contract, or connecting with a workout buddy, start slow by testing your sincerity by regularly engaging in (weekly/daily):

- Park further away in parking lots to force yourself to walk.

- Take the steps when you can.

- Walk the dog that is always looking at you in hopes that you will walk him/her.

- Do chair exercises while sitting: sit up straight in your chair and place your right arm behind your right hip, then twist to the right and hold then do the same on the left and alternate sides. Do side stretches by leaning to one side and then the other, touch your toes while seated by stretching your legs out and bending over.

- Take a lunchtime walk, or walk after dinner.

- Conference calls get boring, we all know that, so while you're on the phone, get up and start walking.

- If public transit is your primary source of transportation, maybe get off the bus a few stops early and walk to your destination.

- When working from home, my cousin walks around her house at lunchtime.

The idea is to start small and stay CONSISTENT with it. If you can do something consistently for a while, you may be ready for one of the bigger commitments mentioned earlier. As a person who is dependent on instruction and motivation for fitness, you need to teach yourself some form of dedication to help you stick with a program.

Man Down—Carry On

If you do team up with a workout partner, be cautious of a non-dedicated buddy. Some want to blame their lack of exercise on a friend not going with them. It is motivating to have a friend to work out with, but this person must be serious. If you absolutely need a partner, do not let their days missed become your days missed. Make a promise to yourself to go solo on the days that your partner misses. If you are uncomfortable being alone, take your headphones.

Nine Ways to Improve Your Consistency in Your Exercise Routine:

1. Getting to the gym or getting your workout routine consistent starts with blocking time out on your calendar and firmly telling yourself that nothing will override the decision. Kind of like the airlines' black-out dates or that coupon you so intended on using for your dinner but the server tells you that it is not honorable on weekends. You cannot argue with her! Stand firm with your "blocked out" dates on your calendar for your workouts. In my opinion, it is all too easy to override exercise time and the guilt is easy to ignore. Changing your willingness to opt-out so easily and increasing your guilt feelings if you miss your workout is key to getting your exercise routine consistent. So, pencil in, mark, or enter your exercise time on your calendar a month or two in advance, just like a doctor's appointment, and stick to it! For me, marking when you plan on working out or marking after you work out on a calendar is helpful. Remember, if you can mark 20 minutes of exercise on a calendar 2 times a week, that is 2,080 minutes of exercise per year, and 4 times a week would be 4,160 minutes of exercise! It adds up fast! Buy a calendar specifically for exercise and hang it somewhere where you can see it. Putting a reminder on your phone might mean you get distracted by your favorite social media site when you pick up your phone!

2. Devices and social media. Too much time on the internet and our favorite social media sinkholes can cause the clock to go very fast and before you know it, five or so things you had hoped to accomplish, weren't accomplished. Make the internet and social media a reward and not a daily habit. After you accomplish your workout, allow yourself to engage on the internet. When I was small, "after you" was very popular, but in today's society, not so much.

After you do your homework
After you clean your room
After you do the dishes

After you walk the dog
After you help your brother
AFTER YOU DO YOUR WORKOUT!

3. Choose your time block wisely. I found that I am more likely to exercise if I get it out of the way early in the morning. This is just the best time for me because I have too many other things that may pop up if I don't. One of the biggest distractions is a bad day at work and the need to go out with friends or just go out to dinner because I am too exhausted to do anything else like cook, walk the dog, or work out. When you know that your workout time competes with other things that may pop up then move the time to a different part of your day. If you have kids or older parents who need your attention, move your workout to when they are least likely to need you.

4. Be cautious of what you do the day before your planned workout. If I do skip the gym, many times it is due to me having to get errands done because I fell behind the day before. So take care of business the day before. **Do not party or stay up late the night before** a planned workout because being tired makes it easier to excuse yourself from the gym. Make going out a reward after you do your workout; don't allow that glass of wine, beer, or favorite beverage until you bang out that workout.

5. Ask people for help to get your exercise mission accomplished. It is very common to ask someone for help when you need to go to the doctor, whether it is to drive you there, go with you, or watch your children, but how often do you hear, "Will you watch my kids while I go to the gym?" or "Can you drive me to the gym?" Going to the gym is just as important as going to the doctor. Exercise sustains your health. Ask your partner to do an errand that pops up on your blackout date; ask a friend or your parents to transport your child to their event. You can always offer to return the favor if they need something. Don't allow pop-ups to get in your way.

6. Television. If television is your excuse, learn to record the shows you watch. Limit the shows that you watch. Move the TV into the room/gym where you work out. Bring the exercise to the living room. Add up the hours that you spend watching TV and reevaluate your priorities.

7. I didn't sleep last night or I'm too tired. On these days, exercising can actually make you feel more energized. It increases your blood flow which pumps oxygen to your brain, muscles, and tissues faster. It also promotes the release of neurotransmitters like dopamine, serotonin, and natural endorphins that will make you feel better and more energetic. Even moderate exercise can improve your energy levels!

Plus, exercise can actually help you sleep better by reducing anxiety and depressive symptoms. It has been proven that exercise reduces these symptoms in the general population. There has not been a lot of research on exercise to determine how much exercise is needed, how it may help with insomnia or getting a better night's sleep, or which exercises are best and what time of day is best. However, with what little research is out there, exercise looks promising to be a contender in helping people get better sleep.

8. Feed your mind with the thoughts of how awesome it feels when you are leaving the gym after completing your workout. You know how good that feels! Promise yourself the luxury of mind and body satisfaction. Be bound and determined to get your workout in for the day so you can enjoy that good mental feeling!

9. Do not be intimidated. As I said, fitness folk are some of the kindest people on earth—they are constantly releasing their happy hormones. Yes, it is tough at first when you are new in a class, in a gym, or on an engaging fitness app, but getting through those beginning stages or the first few times will be very rewarding! You can do it!

The Dependent Person is the most difficult to get moving and stay committed. If you are in this category, you may need a mental push:

Here is your mental push:

A study from the National Cancer Institute published in JAMA Internal Medicine[2] strongly supports the theory that regular exercise reduces the risk of many types of cancers (for both men and women). The research team compared the rates of cancer in those people with the highest levels of physical activity and those with the lowest levels. They found that those with the highest levels of physical activity had lower rates of cancer. Regular exercise leads to changes in the body (like less inflammation, better immune function, and higher levels of natural antioxidants) that reduce the risk of cancer.[3]

Great motivation and reasons to shed the pounds and start getting some fitness in daily!

No matter what type of person you are, independent, slightly independent, or dependent, a consistent fitness plan will be beneficial to your health and is a necessity for maintaining or losing weight. It can be tough trying to develop your routine on your own and sticking with it, but success with this can make a huge difference. Strive to master your own fitness plan! Whatever your excuse is, see it as a wall that you need to get around in a life-or-death situation!

Literature Cited in this Chapter

1. Uberoi R. Gym rat: crowdsourcing personal trainers. Harvard Digital Innovation and Transformation. March 20, 2017. https://d3.harvard.edu/platform-digit/submission/gym-rat-crowdsourcing-personal-trainers/

2. Patel AV, Hildebrand JS, Campbell PT, et al. Leisure-Time spent sitting and Site-Specific cancer incidence in a large U.S. cohort. *Cancer Epidemiology, Biomarkers & Prevention*. 2015;24(9):1350-1359. doi:10.1158/1055-9965.epi-15-0237

3. Does Regular Exercise Reduce Cancer Risk? Harvard Health Publishing. July 12, 2016. https://www.health.harvard.edu/exercise-and-fitness/does-regular-exercise-reduce-cancer-risk

Chapter 21

What To Look for In a Workout App

Before choosing a workout app, check with your doctor or medical provider to verify it is the best one for you. Some workout apps have been around for years, while others come and go. You may not be familiar with how customized workout apps can be. This chapter provides a look at their versatility and what they can offer, so you can make a choice that specifically fits your needs. The apps are organized into categories so you can see some of their specialties although they are not limited to those specialties.

Some people like having accountability, and for this need, some apps have an instructor to see them via video stream. Others prefer no accountability and might be better off with an offline video or an audio coach in their ear. There are workouts for "in-home" and there are ones that involve the outdoors. Whether you're looking for a new HIIT program (*high-intensity interval training)*, marathon-training schedule, 30-day yoga challenge, or daily aerobics routine there are plenty of apps and websites to help you along.

This chapter just provides a look at what some apps may offer and how fun they can be. These apps and their features may change or be discontinued over time. Researching the most current version of these apps and what they offer/provide is highly recommended.

Quick Workouts

The Johnson & Johnson Official 7-Minute Workout app - A circuit-training workout app that lets you squeeze some exercise into your day at an intensity level that's right for you. All you need is a chair and about seven minutes. Some workouts are longer and some are more intense, some less intense. A medium-intensity workout may include jumping jacks, wall chair sits, high-knee running in place, triceps dips on a chair, and a few other moves. Audio and visual cues tell you when to start and stop each exercise and a video demonstration appears in the middle to guide you. The Johnson & Johnson Official 7 Minute Workout app is suitable for just about anyone at any ability level.

Onyx - You can commit to as little as five minutes, or more if you prefer. Onyx brings the workouts to your home. By positioning your phone on the floor and propping it up against the wall, Onyx utilizes your camera to capture and track your reps and watch your form. While the instructor explains and performs the moves (pushups, planks, lunges, etc.) on the screen, your image appears in the upper left-hand corner. The App analyzes your movement, and the trainer explains how you can improve or correct your form.

Sworkit Fitness & Workout app - At-home and on-the-go workout system suited for everyone from beginners to pro-athletes. Whether you're looking to lose weight, tone up, gain muscle, improve your flexibility, or increase your endurance, Sworkit is for you. Providing 5-minute to 45-minute workouts with equipment (Resistance bands, kettlebells, dumbbells) or no equipment workouts.

Workouts on Demand – Watch Pre-Recorded Videos Anytime

For those who like a variety in their routine such as a high-intensity workout one day and an intermediate yoga lesson the next; or bodyweight exercises followed by a stretching session. Some on-demand workout apps coach you through prerecorded videos while others connect you to live classes or coaches via video stream.

Shred - Creates workouts for you to do with some basic equipment you might have at home or in a gym.

The workouts are based on your goals. You may want to solely build muscle or maybe you'd rather blend some cardio into your muscle-building routine. Whatever the case, Shred builds a complete program, so you know what to do and which days to do it. The app suggests the number of repetitions you should do, which you can adjust, and you decide on the weight. If you're looking to build muscle and need help to figure out how to do this, Shred may be perfect for you.

FitOn - Provides follow-along video workouts in a variety of styles, including weight training, stretching and yoga, kickboxing, high-intensity interval cardio (HIIT), boot camp, weightlifting, dance, barre, meditation, and bodyweight classes to work your muscles and challenge users of all fitness levels. New workouts are posted daily.

Keelo - A high-intensity strength and conditioning program that delivers real, measurable fitness results with more than 150 static workouts available and allows you to connect a heart rate monitor during your session. When you browse the App's catalog of workouts, you can see a preview of each session before you start. A workout functional map that tells you which of the various parts of the body will get a workout.

Trainiac - Workout app in which a personal trainer creates workout plans just for you. After completing a short questionnaire about, your fitness level, what equipment you have on hand, your goals, and motivations for working out, Trainiac then suggests personal trainers. You read their profiles to learn more about their areas of specialization and then choose one you'd like to try training with. However, the trainer doesn't coach you through them in real-time. You will receive instructions and videos showing you how to do each exercise.

Live Streaming

Forte. Fit-Forte - A website where you can stream live workout classes and join them from your home, a remote gym, a hotel room, or any place you want to work out. You will see and hear the instructor teaching a real class, but no one sees or hears you. When you browse available classes, you can see the date and time, how long the class will be, how intense it will be, what equipment if any is needed, and other details. Some classes call for nothing more than a mat, while others utilize free weights, stationary bicycles, and more.

Activity Tracking

Activity-tracking apps keep a record of all the activities you do, such as running, bicycle riding, and walking. These apps create a log of all your activities and the stats associated with them, such as how many calories you burned or whether your bicycle ride today was as long as yesterday.

Many activity-tracking apps connect with fitness trackers to make it easier to record your activities. Some include heart rate monitors, too. The heart rate monitor, chest strap or watch, records your heart rate as you move and creates a graph of your heart rate when you finish.

Find What Feels Good - Adriene Mishler has launched an app called Find What Feels Good, or FWFG, which comes from a line she uses when reminding fellow yoga students to adjust their postures according to their bodies. FWFG has single-session yoga, a series of practices that you can do across many days, and a calendar for keeping track of your progress.

FitOn: Fitness Workout Plans Workouts on demand that you can find based on how much time you have, the level of intensity that you want, or the type of workout you're hoping to do (yoga, glutes, and thighs, abs, stretching, etc.). If you wear a connected heart rate monitor while working out, you can see your heart rate on the screen while you follow the video. There's also a leaderboard where you can compete with other members or a group of friends.

Jefit – Used to plan and track your workouts. It comes with a customizable workout planner, an abundant exercise library, and a members-only Facebook group. You can choose new workouts and track your progress. It keeps you on track to see how close you are to reaching your fitness goals.

Apps That Require At-Home Exercise Equipment

Peloton - An at-home exercise bike that features a large screen on the front and rear speakers, allowing you to work out to one of the thousands of classes available through the Peloton All-Access membership.

Tonal - Tonal is a large, rectangular, wall-mounted device that displays interactive workout programming on a big screen. A pair of adjustable arms that extend from the system with a cable that provides an adjustable amount of resistance of up to 100 pounds per arm. Attachable accessories that are included allow you to perform a wide range of strength-building movements, if you desire, from bench presses and squats to bicep curls and rope extensions.

Lululemon Studio Mirror -The Lululemon Studio Mirror fits into any room in your home. When it's off, it's a beautifully designed full-length mirror. When it's on, it's a complete fitness studio with over 10,000 workouts and over 50 class types, taught by the nation's top instructors via the Lululemon Studio App.

Workout Music Apps

For those who love music, research has shown that listening to music can reduce anxiety, blood pressure, and pain as well as improve sleep quality, mood, mental alertness, and memory.

FIT Radio

Fit Radio is a music-streaming app that also has playlists for guided workouts. Whether you want workout music selected by DJs or a voice in your ear encouraging you to pick up the pace on your treadmill. Fit Radio has songs/genres that fit the type of workout you enjoy. FIT Radio can introduce you to **new music** with a beat that matches your workout, whether it's CrossFit, running, Zumba, or yoga.

RockMyRun - Customize your workouts with professional DJ-caliber mixing, songs that match your running tempo, or tracks made for your activity of choice, such as elliptical training or yoga.

It can find your heartbeat with a connected heart rate monitor or detect your footfalls while you run and then find songs from a wide variety of genres with the right tempo.

Exercise and Diet Combined

8fit - Combines various on-demand workout videos and meal planning. The app creates a personalized program for your diet and exercise based on your goals. It benefits people who like a lot of guidance, suggestions, reminders, and instructions. You choose a goal, whether it is to lose weight, tone your body, or gain muscle. Then you make your goal more specific, like decreasing body fat to 20% in three months. 8fit takes into consideration a lot of details about you when designing your fitness plan, such as what time of day you exercise. It provides a customized shopping list to your tastes for meal plans and you can log what you eat.

Centr - Australian actor Chris Hemsworth, brings you this all-in-one fitness app for planning your training, workouts, and healthy eating. You can use it to build muscle, lose weight, or get fit by telling the app which of these goals you're interested in during the signup process.

Fitbit Coach - Personalized training app motivates you to reach your health and fitness goals, learn how to improve your nutrition, get stronger, and lose a few pounds with expert-designed dynamic bodyweight, run, and walk workouts that continually adjust to your feedback, goals, and capabilities. At home or traveling you can get a great workout anytime, anywhere like you have a personal trainer right there with you.

Jillian Michaels Fitness app - Combines workouts and meal planning for a well-rounded wellbeing and fitness experience. Celebrity and expert trainer Jillian Michaels is your coach through every workout. You watch her on screen and listen to her encouragement to finish each exercise. Everything about the app is customizable, from the foods you get in your meal suggestions to the types of workouts for you. You also rate workouts as easy, medium, or hard so that they continually stay challenging at your fitness level. This program might be a little intense for people who are not already somewhat fit. It's great for anyone looking to drop a few pounds and gain some muscle.

Openfit - User-friendly online wellness app offering live classes in which the certified trainers can see you and provide feedback in real-time. They cheer you on, keep you motivated, and can help improve your form with video instruction. Plus, a large variety of on-demand exercise videos and programs and the option to opt into meal plans and nutritional tracking all from the comfort of your home.

Competitive

Strava - Fitness-tracking app for runners, cyclists, and swimmers who are seeking a bit of competition. In Strava you compete against yourself or other people who have also run, biked, or swam the same segments that you have. The app uses the GPS from your phone or a connected device to track exactly where you go and how fast. Then it analyzes your data and your competitors to see where you overlapped to compute a segment leaderboard for all.

Map My Fitness – This is one of the best exercise-tracking apps for people who are beginners. It has hundreds of activities you can track, from vacuuming to rock climbing. You will see how even daily activities can add up to a fitter lifestyle. Any time you're about to do an activity, you launch the App, choose the activity, and start recording. The app will tell you how much time you spend doing it, calories burned, as well as other stats that change based on what you're doing. You can compete with other members and claim your spot at the top of the leaderboard. Each challenge comes with different activities, rules, and prizes!

Charity Miles - It motivates you by donating funds to the organization of your choice for every mile you run, walk, or bicycle when you use the app to log the miles. Corporate sponsors agree to donate a few cents for every mile you complete, and in exchange, you see their advertising and information about them in the App. Charity Miles supports many nonprofit organizations, such as ASPCA, Habitat for Humanity, St. Jude Children's Hospital, UNICEF, Save the Children, and the Wounded Warrior Project. Knowing that your activity supports charitable causes may just motivate you to move every day.

CHAPTER 22

Injury/Health Issues and Exercise

Working Out During an Injury

The purpose of this chapter is not to educate you on working out, treating injuries, or determining if you have an injury. The purpose of this chapter is to inform you that you should always try to keep moving if you want to avoid weight gain and diabetes. I often hear people say that they used to exercise; but now, because of an injury or health issue, they no longer can. Is your issue really a serious injury or is it an excuse to not exercise? An injury or condition is not an excuse to take a break from your health and fitness routine unless it is very serious. Any type of movement will burn calories, reduce blood sugar, and have mental benefits.

Even with an injury, you can continue exercising; you just need to modify your routine and get creative. For example, if you have a lower-body injury, an upper-body and core workout could be possible. These types of workouts include arm bike, weightlifting, chin-ups/pull-ups, curls, triceps dips, bench presses, overhead presses, rowing, and waist twists/bends to name a few. Swimming takes the pressure off your knees and may also be a good fit. If you have an upper-body injury, work your lower body by walking, running, biking, stationary bike, leg raises, and or squats. If you can't walk, run, or bike, go to the pool. There are so many options and there is really no excuse for you to put your exercise routine on hold. Work around your pain and think of it as a fun opportunity to work on a different part of your body while your injured part heals. Stay positive and you can still make progress, even while injured. Research suggests that maintaining a positive, upbeat attitude during an injury or issue can help speed up the healing process.

Serious Injuries/Issues

If you do work out regularly then you may know that it is no fun to try to work out when you are in pain. If your injury is serious, such as a muscle pull or strain, sprained ankle, shoulder injury, knee injury, shin splint, tendinitis, arthritis, wrist sprain, or dislocation, **it is most important that you first see a doctor for proper evaluation and instructions.** It is okay to train through pain, but it is never okay to train through a serious injury. So, if you are seriously injured, see a doctor right away before it turns into a chronic problem or gets worse. The doctor may give you a resting time which you should follow. The consequences of continuing to train when you have a serious injury and not taking enough time off to heal can be severe. If you re-injure your body, it may take longer to heal the second time. So, for a severe injury, take the time to let it heal. However, after your resting time, explain to the doctor that you would like to continue exercising and ask what you can do and when you can start. The doctor may NOT provide this information unless you ask. For this chapter, I interviewed and received a wealth of knowledge from Theresa Ivancik IFBB Pro (International Federation of Bodybuilding) 4x Professional Champion, 3x Olympian, fitness model, Certified Personal Trainer and entrepreneur. Theresa said,

> Occasionally what doctors will discuss with you could end up limiting you, by responding with an answer that you don't want to hear. I see this on numerous occasions, where the client then becomes unmotivated. This is where I think a lot of people just give up or steer away from exercise, but the work can still be done. The person knows their body and how they want to live the rest of their life. Exercise and mobility will help you heal faster and possibly live longer. Do not be afraid to talk to your doctor and discuss the things that are important to you. If you do not ask, you might not receive any suggestions for other ways to exercise during your injury. An injury and/or health problem can make it difficult to exercise, but if you are truly interested in an exercise routine to benefit your health, ask this question and tell your doctor that you really want and need to exercise. A sedentary lifestyle has no benefits.

How a Certified Personal Trainer Can Help

Theresa has trained people with serious injuries as well as cancer, diabetes, heart disease, and dementia. She said,

"Many people do not realize that you can ask your doctor to connect with your Certified Personal Trainer. They will most likely be happy to work together to help you get better, but you have to ask." A quality Certified Personal Trainer may offer more than a physical therapist who may just help with your initial rehabilitation therapy at a rehab center. The benefits of a Certified Personal Trainer are:

1. They work muscle groups that expand to ALL muscles involved in your injury.

2. They will also know how to do your usual exercises with isolation, so the injured muscle is not used. This is helpful with injuries like a rotator cuff or shoulder and knee replacement.

3. They are more likely to stand right beside you, and not walk away, to monitor and assist with imploring correct procedure. They help with stability and range of motion when working out.

Theresa explained a couple of examples of working out with an injury. The first was for a knee replacement and using isolation movements.

> You can hold on to a Smith machine bar, or even a table in your house to perform a one-leg squat with the good leg so it can remain strong and take the pressure and the slack from having the injury. This will help repair the injured leg as well. I would recommend, if possible, going into surgery as fit and healthy as you can, this will ensure faster healing and muscle strength. During the healing phase, to regain strength, it is important to work the muscle groups together and also isolated. Body weight squats are a great way to start, then moving into a one-leg squat or one leg press holding onto a bar or light weight.
>
> Leg extensions and hamstring curls are also two very good machines that can control your range of motion and the weight you use. Be sure to do both legs together, but also do isolation as well. Using an aerobic step can also be beneficial, use at the lowest height you can, then slowly increase the height each week.

Assuming that you have already been to a doctor/hospital for your injury, make a list of exercises that you enjoy and think you could do that would not impact your injury/issue. Take this list to a Certified Personal Trainer to get the ball rolling. You might think that a Personal Trainer sounds expensive but, in my experience, Personal Trainers are some of the kindest people I have ever met, and they may provide some free advice if you stop by a local gym. You could also reach out to a high-school athletic director. Take their suggestions and information to your doctor for approval. Then you will be consulting with two professionals. A second opinion is always valuable; your health and safety are worth it!

Your doctor may refer you to a physical therapist. Having both a Certified Personal Trainer and a physical therapist and having them communicate on your behalf with the doctor would be ideal. Having three consultants is fine!

Working Out with a Chronic Disease

Heart disease — Aerobic exercise and interval training can help improve your heart health and aid with weight loss.

Diabetes — Exercise can help lower blood sugar levels, maintain weight, and boost your energy. If you have Type 2 diabetes, exercise can lower your risk of heart disease.

Asthma — Exercise can control the frequency and severity of asthma attacks.

Back pain — Regular low-impact aerobic exercises or yoga can increase strength and endurance and improve muscle function in your back. Abdominal and back muscle exercises (core-strengthening exercises) may help reduce symptoms by strengthening the muscles around your spine.

Cancer — Exercise can improve your mood.

Dementia — Exercise can improve cognition and cognitive impairment in people with dementia.

As mentioned earlier, Theresa Ivancik trains clients with chronic diseases such as diabetes, thyroid disease, fibromyalgia, and breast cancer, and she has seen their progress and improvements. Exercise might limit the impact of Type 2 diabetes by reducing the number of insulin shots, eliminating thyroid medicine, and even losing over 100 pounds, these have been some of the results of her training and dietary advice to her clients. She trained a female client who had a serious atrial fibrillation issue.

> She was not authorized by her doctor to do any strength training and to only do light cardio activity ...... really limiting her capabilities. With the help of Garmin Heart Rate Monitors, she was allowed to train with me. I stood beside her during her training. Her heart got stronger and received more oxygen. Strength training increases chances of surviving heart conditions."

After training with Theresa, she is now doing 100% strength training, bodybuilding competitions and even snow skiing.

How Nutrition Can Play a Part in Avoiding and Healing from Injuries

Theresa also told me that proper nutrition and anti-inflammatory foods can help with reducing inflammation around your injury and this is an additional step that may help your recovery. One of the most important factors in injury recovery that can dramatically accelerate the healing process is to get adequate nutrition. Healing is greatly dependent on blood supply, and the stronger the blood supply, the faster you can heal. Blood supplies the injured area with oxygen and nutrients which assist the injury in healing. Certain foods can promote inflammation within the body, while others have an anti-inflammatory effect. Avoid inflammation-promoting foods such as fried foods and processed white flour. Eat more foods that are high in omega-3 fatty acids. Fish (especially mackerel), green vegetables, wild rice, Pecans, cod liver oil, flaxseeds, walnuts, salmon, chia seeds, cold-pressed olive oil, pumpkin seeds, soybeans, eggs, sardines, spinach, papaya, Brussels sprouts, oysters, anchovies, and caviar. These foods contain omega-3 fatty acids which are extremely beneficial and are an integral part of cell membranes throughout the body. They affect the function of the cell receptors in these membranes. Omega-3 fatty acids help with hormone production; they regulate blood clotting, contraction, and relaxation of artery walls and levels of inflammation in the body. A diet of processed foods, fried foods, soda, and sugar will provide no such help in the healing process.

Drink a lot of water and replace soda with plenty of fresh juices made from fresh, organic, raw veggies, because raw veggies are high in important enzymes and vitamins that can speed up the healing process—garlic, radishes, and beets are especially helpful. Fresh ginger has powerful anti-inflammatory properties that help reduce pain and soreness. Eat 8–10 servings of fruit and vegetables daily for best results.

In addition, you might ask your doctor about other nutrients and vitamins that might aid in tissue repair and provide you with other health benefits.

Important Vitamins and Nutrients That May Aid in Tissue Repair

Before taking any of these vitamins or nutrients, please remember to ask your doctor or nutritionist if they might be helpful to you.

Multivitamin: Very important. Helps prevent vitamin and mineral deficiencies.

Zinc: Important in tissue repair.

Vitamin C with bioflavonoids: An important antioxidant that helps tissue repair and growth.

Manganese: Strengthens wounded tendons and ligaments.

Amino acids: (BCAA): Helps promote the healing of muscle tissue, bones, and skin.

Essential fatty acids: Speed up recovery and promote cellular health.

Vitamin B complex: Helps reduce injury-related stress.

Glucosamine sulfate: Helps strengthen and form tendons, cartilage, ligaments, and joint fluid.

Calcium: Helps repair connective tissue.

Silica complex: Important for memory and connective tissue of the brain. Also, it is unbeatable for bone building and bone protection and is crucial for bone/joint repair and recovery.

For Non-Injured People

If you currently do not have an injury or disease and have no problems with exercising, do everything in your power to avoid an injury/issue!

Steps You Can Take to Avoid Getting Injured

Some of this information can be found in Jamin Thompson's "10 Tips for Injury Work-Arounds" which can be found at http://www.bodybuilding.com/fun/10-tips-when-training-with-an-injury.html.[1]

1. ALWAYS WARM UP PROPERLY

Having a warm-up routine to get your body ready for exercise, which will gradually increase your heart rate, is very beneficial and will also loosen your muscles and joints. If you quickly flex or place tension on a cold muscle, you increase your risk of injury to that muscle. But if you gradually raise the temperature of the muscle and then slowly stretch it out with "static stretching" (to stretch and hold a muscle in a *comfortable* position for a period, usually 10 to 30 seconds) it will help relax and elongate the muscle, and place it in an injury-resistant state. This is also a great bonus for your state of mind before working out as happy hormones are released when you stretch and exercise.

A proper warm-up is really important!

2. If you have not exercised in a while, ease into it, don't push yourself too hard or try to achieve what you used to do.

For example, as a child, you may have been fond of swinging from a rope and falling into the water. Our body changes weight-wise; our weight shifts and our upper body may not be able to support our weight like it used to. Grabbing onto a rope swing as an adult could be dangerous because you may have to let go before you are over the water. If you were once a snow skier on black diamond hills, you would be wise to start on green hills if you have not skied in a while. Your legs may not be able to brace for the impact.

3. Use proper form to avoid injury and accidents

Whether you are playing volleyball, swimming, running, weight-lifting, or riding a bike, it is always a good idea to consult with a person who is a professional in that category and gain knowledge of proper form. A common reason for injuries is a failure to use proper form. There is a proper way to hit a golf ball, ski, lift weights, run/jog, do yoga, etc. Take the time to learn the proper ways and correct procedures for whatever type of exercise you are doing because the incorrect technique can place your muscles, tendons, and joints in unnatural positions and increase the likelihood of an injury such as a muscle or tendon tear. Keep in mind that your limbs can only move in certain ways; and contorting, jerking, or twisting can result in an injury. The human body has very specific biomechanical pathways that we must adhere to if we want to remain injury-free.

4. Improper procedures or not learning proper safety

Being unfamiliar with rules can also place you in harm's way for accidents, such as not knowing safety rules for riding a real bike on the road and possibly being struck by a vehicle. Running or jogging along the road can be dangerous as well. Learn about and follow signs when biking, hiking, skiing, climbing, and other outdoor sports. Listen to instructions and read any materials provided.

5. Cool Down

Post-workout, a cooldown period of 5–10 minutes will help slowly bring your heart rate, breathing, and body temperature back to normal. Focus on deep breathing and stretching the muscles that were just used. This can prevent fainting and dizziness and can prevent the immediate post-exercise tendency for muscle spasms or cramping. Stretching both before and after exercise will increase flexibility and may help prevent injury. Cooling down can also reduce muscle soreness and stiffness.

Post-Injury Return Rules

No Pain, No Problem? Your injury may have not required you to go to a doctor or you just didn't go to a doctor but don't return too quickly to your regular routine once the pain is gone. This is a very common mistake many people make post-injury. Once your pain starts to go away, you might jump back into the routine where you endured the injury, which can cause a re-injury. It will take time to rebuild your muscle tissue. Just because the pain is gone, does not mean that the muscle is ready for the same routine/exercise you did before. Using an injured muscle too quickly can not only cause a re-injury, but it may take longer to heal the second time. Be very cautious with how hard you push yourself. This is the same for someone who is trying a new exercise. Ease into it because you probably will be using muscles that you haven't used in a while.

In conclusion, be careful to avoid an injury. If you do get injured, see a doctor and possibly a physical therapist. It is extra helpful to consult with a Certified Personal Trainer for help to heal and exercise through your injury. Take care of your injury so you heal properly and quickly. Eat anti-inflammatory foods and stay away from fast food and ultra-processed foods. The worst choice to make when you are injured or have a health issue is to become sedentary and say goodbye to exercise. Work your other healthy muscles to stay in exercise mode and don't let an injury or health issue become your EXCUSE.

Literature Cited in this Chapter

1. Thompson J. 10 Tips for injury work-arounds. July 2, 2020. https://www.bodybuilding.com/content/10-tips-when-training-with-an-injury.html

CHAPTER 23

45 Super-Fun Non-Technology Activities for Kids

Keep in mind that I am the Mom of two girls, so many of these activities are female-oriented. However, this should provide ideas for you to create your own fun and activities for your kids whether they are boys or girls. You can customize these activities to fit your kids' gender and passions. The idea is to get your kids moving and not just sitting and staring at their phones or the television. Each activity listed has a brief description before it: how many kids can play, what age group, items needed, what season, indoors or outside, prep time, and possible problems. Some activities are listed as "physical" just to note that they were strong allies in helping reduce blood sugar. This chapter will provide all you need to pre-plan activities to do/play with your kids, making it quick and easy for when it is playtime.

Also, relative words are in bold for you to share terminology while playing with your kids to educate them! It is never too early to start prepping them for school and the standardized testing that schools require. Kids love to learn in a fun environment and introducing them to new terms and new concepts that match the activity is always fun and stimulating for their minds. At the end of each activity, there is a favorite memory from my kids!

Disclaimer: You or your child's participation in any of the activities in this book is at your sole and exclusive risk. Injuries and damages can occur by natural causes or by the acts of other persons or third parties, either as a result of negligence or because of other reasons. All activities require parental supervision at all times.

Note: The ages and number of players are just suggestions, as well as all other information. These activities are open to any gender and can be customized to fit any child's interests.

1. Balloon Volleyball — A favorite! (physical)

Players: 2–8
Age: 2 and up
Items needed: Balloon or beach ball
Season: Any — but great for an indoor activity in the winter
Indoor/Outdoor
Prep time: 2 minutes — blow up a balloon and if playing indoors, move furniture to create a safe space to play.
Possible problems: If you are using a beach ball you may want to move any delicate objects out of the way.
Favorite memory from my kids: "My favorite game! We hit the balloon for hours!"

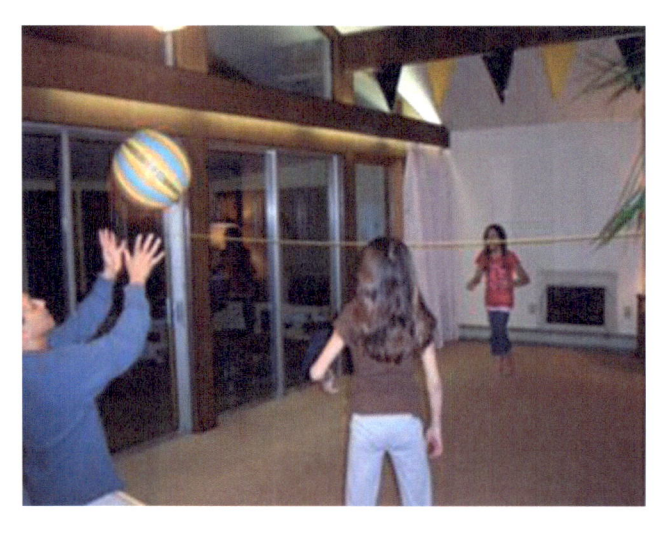

2. Chemist/Laboratory

Players: 2–4
Age: 6 to 12
Items needed: Pitcher of water, food coloring, **test tubes, liquid medicine dispensers, measuring cups**, little medicine measuring cups, clear plastic cups, measuring spoons, a table, and old T-shirts or a plastic smock to protect clothing.
Season: Summer and outdoor is best because it can be messy.
Indoor/Outdoor

Prep time: Possibly 30 minutes to set up a table and gather items. You may have to order or buy a few items depending on how much you want to simulate a laboratory.

Possible problems: Can be messy.

For those with little kids, you most likely have little medicine cups that come with children's liquid medicine. This all started because we have a pool, and we had a PH **chemical monitoring test kit**. They used to watch their dad test the pool's chemical balance for too much **acidity or alkalinity.** We had an old kit and I would give my daughters food coloring and a pitcher of water for them to make colors in the tester. This is a great way to show them how mixing colors creates new colors. You can order play test tubes or a play chemistry kit online ahead of time. **Teach them about the mix, stir, strain, beaker, tongs, crucible, funnel, forceps, graduated cylinder, mortar and pestle, spatula, stirring rod, test tube, thermometer, chemistry, formulas, laboratory tools, glassware, equipment, science, composition, combustion, structure, matter, atoms, chemical reactions, chemical compounds.**

Favorite memory from my kids: "It was cool to use the test kit that Dad always tested the pool water with."

3. Couch Pool (adult needed—use caution)

Players: 1–6
Age: 3–10
Items needed: Couch and couch cushions, lots of pillows and blankets
Season: Summer or winter
Indoors
Prep time: 5 minutes
Possible problems: Kids are too tired to help clean up! Tell your little ones they have to help put the blanket and pillows away.

If you have more than one child, make sure that they jump one at a time and make sure they wait until the previous jumper gets out of the pool. This one always shocked the neighbors' kids when they saw that we were actually jumping off of our couch into a pile of pillows on the floor. If you have a sectional sofa, great, just arrange all the cushions on the floor in the middle and top with extra pillows and cover with a blanket to hold the pillows together. Make sure any sharp-edge furniture is not near and let the kids jump from the couch into the center where all the pillows are. I would recommend watching the little ones with this activity to make sure they are only jumping into the pillows. For those without a sectional, it may be more difficult to keep all the pillows together. Use other soft furniture such as recliners or ottomans to surround the pillows. This is a great mid-winter evening exercise and the kids really do enjoy it! You can ask the older kids to be "**lifeguards**" and watch that the younger kids are following the rules. You can have a deeper end (more pillows) and explain that this is the deep side because of the **depth**. There can be a swim-up bar where swimmers can get a drink of water. This is also a great way to demonstrate the **breaststroke**, the **butterfly**, **side-stroke**, and **backstroke**. This is an opportunity to teach **pool safety** to your children and show them how to throw a **flotation device** (a pillow) to someone who is drowning in the pool of pillows.

Teach them about drowning, distressed swimmers, heat exhaustion, CPR, aquatic facilities, rescue, filters, chlorine, skimmers, pool cleaners, and vacuums.

Favorite memory from my kids: "Going under the loose blanket and pretending that we were underwater."

4. Create a Magazine

Players: 1–4
Age: 5–16
Items needed: Paper, scissors, tape, stapler, crayons or markers, newspapers, rubber cement, magazines/newspapers, pen, ruler, any helpful art supplies, stapler
Season: Any
Indoor
Prep time: 15 minutes to gather items
Possible problems: We never had any problems.

Ask your kids to create a magazine! Help them put blank pages together with staples and tell them to create a magazine name and a **cover page**. Help them number the pages and create a **table of contents**. See what kind of ideas they come up with and help them put their creativity into a magazine!!! Tell them about **bar codes and ISBNs**, and list the **editors, photographers, writers**, etc. Determine a **price. Teach them about print, printer, publication, headline, banner, binding, sheets, margins, bleed marks, body text, camera-ready, layout, color separation, column, copy, editorial, feature, centerfold, ads, the masthead, contents, logo, page, paper stock, prepress, final proof, saddle-stitching, spine, spread, stock images, trim, white space.**

Favorite memory from my kids: "I still have one!!!! That was really fun, and we got to cut up other magazines and draw and create fashions."

5. Dance (physical)

Players: 1 to a small group
Age: 2 and up
Items needed: Music and a space to dance. You can add lighting, outfits, costumes
Season: Any
Indoor/Outdoor weather permitting
Prep time: 5 to 15 minutes
Possible problems: Kids may get tired from dancing.

This activity may not last that long, so if you have some decorations and a good imagination, ask the kids if they want to decorate the dance hall. Spending time decorating keeps them moving as well. This is a good time to introduce them to all kinds of music. Ask them if they can dance to Country, Rock, Electronic Dance Music, Rhythm and Blues, Disco, etc. Ask them which one they like the best or which is easiest to dance to. Have a different **genre** each day or a day of the week or one day can be dance day. The kids can dress for the type of music that will be played. Teach them about famous **dancers, different types and eras** of **music, waltz, tango, cha-cha-cha-, rumba, samba, mambo, jive, bolero, swing, Charleston, tap, moonwalk, boogie-woogie, salsa, flamenco, polka, folk, belly, ballet, contemporary, ceremonial, jazz, modern, hip-hop, line, Irish, wedding dances.**

Favorite memory from my kids: "We loved dancing in the basement with socks on because the floor was slippery. We dressed up in costumes! The 80s were the most fun because we teased our hair, wore leotards, and lots of black!"

6. Day-Care Center

Players: 2–4
Age: 3–8
Items needed: Dolls or stuffed animals, doll clothes, play food, play bottles, play pacifiers, toys, coloring books, books, notebook, pen, telephone (pretend), coffee table or any kind of table, child's chair
Season: Summer or winter
Indoor/Outdoor
Prep time: 10 minutes

Possible problems: Kids may argue over who will be the check-in attendant. If you're the mom dropping off a pet or doll, you have to drop them off many times because they love the checking-in process!

To set up for day-care center you will want to try to make a closed-in area. We did this with our couch, coffee table, and a wall. You have to leave an open space to get into the daycare center. If you have one child, you can have either of you sit behind the coffee table (front desk) to **check in** the dolls (babies) that are being dropped off (if you are playing pet-care center, it will be a pet). One player will be in charge of operating the day-care center. Then the other player/s will be the parent or mom dropping off the doll or pet. A notepad or sign-in form will be on the front desk. Tell your kids that they have to ask the questions to complete the form when someone drops them off. Create a form ahead of time with the **parent's name, child's name, contact info, drop-off and pick-up time, cell phone number, emergency contact phone number, doctor's phone number, feeding, or any special instructions**. This is a great way to teach them how to tell the **time and complete a form**. If you have more than one child, there can be an **attendant** taking care of the dolls or pets in the **center** as well as a **check-in** person. Always let your kids give the place a name such as "Daisy's Daycare Center". I would drop off a pet and go to the kitchen to get some things done and my kids always liked to pretend to call me to ask me questions about my doll or pet, like "Does she like to read stories" or "Can she go for a walk."

Favorite memory from my kids: "We got to be real moms!"

7. Ding Ding (physical)

Players: 1–6
Age: 2–5
Items needed: A big circle area to run – this can be a path through the house
Season: Summer or winter
Indoors or outdoors
Prep time: Zero, unless you have to clear an area
Possible problems: None

This activity is for toddlers that can walk fast or run. Shortly after my oldest daughter learned to walk, we started this activity. All she wanted to do was walk. We lived in a split-level home where you could walk through the kitchen into the dining room then through the living room, and back through the kitchen in a circle. We would hold her hand and

take her around and around. When she was able to run, she liked to run through this circle. I would sit in a chair in the living room and every time she came by I would say, "Ding, ding" like she was crossing a **finish line** or finishing a lap. It's extra fun if you have a flag to wave as they come around. Honestly, this was one of the simplest and most fun activities! Her grandfather once took her around 38 times holding her hand when she first started walking—so counting is fun. This activity continued after my second daughter was old enough to walk. They would laugh so hard as I said "Ding, ding." Teach them about the **start, finish, laps, track, pit stops, momentum, leader, and flags.**
Favorite memory from my kids: "That was so fun; it would really get my heart pumping!!"

8. Play Medical Kit

Players: 2–4
Age: 4–8
Season: Summer or winter
Indoors
Prep time: Purchase a play hospital or first aid kit or use what you have in your home—Adhesive bandage, ace bandage, medical tape, gauze, empty pill bottles, play scissors, thermometer, little medicine cups, paper for prescriptions and sign-in sheet, clipboard, pen.
Possible problems: We never really had too many problems with this activity except not enough people to play.
Set up an area in your home with a couple of chairs for the waiting room and use a couch or bed as the examination place. A notepad to write prescriptions and a sign-in notebook and pen. Most kids have been to the **doctor** or school **nurse** so let them use their imagination but you can help them out with learning some **terms like** a **thermometer, temperature, fever, blood pressure, X-ray, prescription, antibiotics, vaccine, influenza, cough syrup, nose spray, Band-Aid, heart rate, cast, sling, etc.** Teach them how to explain what is wrong.
Favorite memory from my kids: "I loved the blue plastic doctor coats made out of trash bags!" (They were art smocks purchased at an arts and crafts store.)

9. Dolls in the Sink

Players: Usually no more than two
Age: 5–8 years old
Items needed: Kitchen sink (double-sided works well for two kids), dolls, trays to put the dolls on when they are wet, dish soap, plastic for the floor, towels, chairs to stand on if using the kitchen sink, dolls, figurines (that can get wet and dry), and any other doll accessories that may be fun to play pretend pool or bath with the dolls.
Season: Any season

Indoors
Prep time: 5 minutes to find items
Possible problems: Water getting all over.
My girls would fill the sink up, put soap in it, and make it a bubble bath for their dolls. This kept them busy for hours, and I am not really sure why!
If you have boys, you can use any figurines or superheroes as **scuba divers**. Teach them spa terms: **aqua aerobics, spa, detoxification, exfoliation, facial, herbal wrap, hot stone therapy, Jacuzzi, loofah scrub, floral bath, medi-spa, mineral spring, whirlpool, sauna.**
You can also teach them environmental terms such as **lagoon/swamp, aquatic, wetland, beach, algae, brook, stream, channel, coast, conservation, lake, flood, drought, well, ditch, basin, floating, habitat, drain, marsh, oasis, pond, puddle, sea, sea level, tide, waterfall, flotation.**
Favorite memory from my kids: "When we turned out the lights and put the night light on and filled the sink with lots of bubbles—we couldn't find the dolls in the sink!"

10. Dress-up 1980s Style (can use any era)

Players: 1–3, or as many as you think you have outfits for
Age: 5 and up
Items needed: A brush or comb to tease hair, leggings or tights, high heels, flashy colors and jewelry
Season: Summer or winter
Indoors
Prep time: This is a planned event; you will have to search for clothing and accessories. Search on the internet for ideas.
You don't have to stick with the 80s, you can teach kids about any era and show them the styles and dress like them. Definitely take a lot of pictures!!! **Teach them about eras, decades, trends, fashion, history,**

styles, timelines, collections, lines, fashion design, designers, couturiers
Possible problems: None.

11. Dress-Up—Runway Model

Players: 1–4 is ideal; we had more at birthday parties
Age: 2–10
Items needed: A long straight area for the **runway**, clothes, jewelry, shoes, hats, make-up (optional), music, dressing room, and chairs along the runway for mom or dad and whoever may be watching the runway show. Camera/phone to take pics.
Season: Winter indoor runway and summer indoor or **outside runway**
Prep time: It can take a while to determine a runway area, set up chairs, and gather clothing and accessories.
Possible problems: Clean-up can be hefty.
This was a favorite of my kids and the outfits that they would put together were priceless memories! Definitely take pictures!!! This can make lifelong memories for your kids and their cousins and or friends. Teach them **fashion industry** terms: **trends, trending, designer, fashion statement, accessories, couture, spring, summer, fall, and winter seasonal fashions, vintage, modeling, photographers, high-fashion models, major fashion markets—New York, Paris, Milan, Tokyo**. If you have boys, and they are not interested in modeling, they can be **clothing designers, photographers, security guards,** or **limo drivers. Get creative**!
Favorite memory from my kids: "Walking the runway after I was dressed in a cool outfit with plastic jewelry and plastic children's heels!"

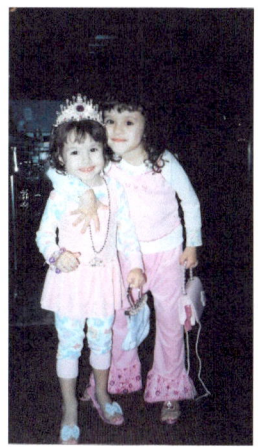

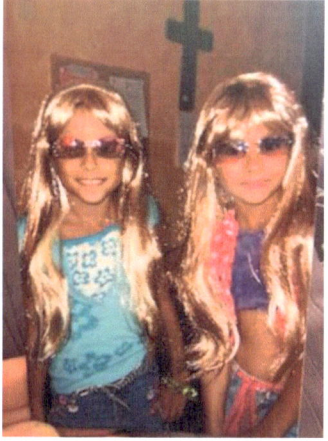

12. Dry-Cleaner

Players: 2–4
Age: 4–10
Items needed: Clothes rack or broomstick and two chairs, tablet, chip clips, coffee table, couch, play money or real money, cash register, box or plastic container to put money in, clothes and lots of hangers, laundry basket(s), play credit card, pen or pencil, a book, small container, note pad, play telephone or cell phone
Season: Summer or winter
Indoors
Prep time: 10 minutes
Possible Problems: Kids may sometimes argue over who is going to perform which job. Clean-up can be intense.

To set up for this activity you will need a room with a little space. If you do not have a clothes rack you can use two chairs and a broomstick to hang hangers with clothes on. You can use a couch for space to put folded clothes on. A coffee table works well as the front desk. If you don't have a cash register, you can use a plastic food container or box. Cut thick paper to make charge cards or use expired real ones. You'll need a notepad for giving receipts and chip clips to attach a ticket to the clothes. Explain the number process to keep track of the clothing. The laundry basket will be for the clothes being dropped off and the small container will be for the receipts when the clothes are picked up.

My kids always liked to operate the dry-cleaning service store (the employee) and I would be the customer dropping off the **garments**. When the customer drops clothes off, the employee will have to take the clothes off the hangers and attach a **numbered ticket** to the clothes with a chip clip. Then the customer will get a **receipt** with the same number on it. If you want to include **coupons** you can make them ahead of time and present them when the clothes are dropped off. The employee will then put the unclean clothes into the laundry basket. If you have multiple kids then another can take the clothes and start the **dry-cleaning process**. We used a second laundry basket to "pretend" to hand wash the clothes in, then shake them dry, and then **iron** them with a book. The garment will then need to be hung up and all buttons, snaps, or zippers closed. **Collars** and or **cuffs** will need special attention. If there are any **spots**, **stains** or damage, or **buttons** that need to be replaced the employee will have to make the repairs and decide if there is an extra charge or not. When the customer's **wardrobe** is complete the garments will have to be **delivered (free delivery)** or picked up. The employee can call the customer to let them know that their wardrobe is ready. Be creative and show your kids what it really might be like to work at or own a dry-cleaner store.

Playing dry cleaner is educational and fun for the kids. Teach them about clothing care, tickets, and how receipts work. Since there are a lot of "props" involved in this activity, make sure that your little ones promise to help clean up.

Favorite memory from my kids: "When we played 'Dry Cleaner' Mom broke out the lint shaver!"

13. Dry Erase Board/ Hangman

Players: 1–5
Age: 5 plus
Items needed: Paper, pen or dry erase board and dry erase marker and eraser
Season: Summer or winter
Outdoors or indoors
Prep time: Just find some paper and a pen or a dry-erase board, a marker, and an eraser. If the paper is taped to the wall, it provides more exercise as they have to get up to draw/play.
Possible problems: None

Ask the kids to try to guess the word you've chosen by guessing one letter at a time. When they guess a correct letter, you put it in the correct space. If they guess a letter and it is incorrect then you draw a part of the hangman. There are videos on YouTube to demonstrate how to play. Teach them about **games, playing, words, phrases, sentences, letters, puzzles, solving, winning, losing, spelling,** and **predicting.**

Favorite memory from my kids: "My Mom and Dad would make the words really funny!"

14. Drive-Through

Players: 2–10
Age: 3 plus
Items needed: Create a window**,** paper or notepad, pen or pencil, plastic cups, plates bowls. Added accessories could be food to play with, a headset, fake money, fake credit cards, a hat, or a **bell**! (they love the bell!)
Season: Summer or winter
Outdoors or indoors
Prep time: 5 to 10 minutes

Possible problems: Some kids want to always be the person taking orders, writing on the pad, and preparing the food to hand through the window.

Drive-through is so fun for the kids. It seems that the kids all want to be taking the orders and getting the food ready, so I went through the "drive-through" a lot of times! When the kids are little they like to see you pretend to eat the food! I always had a very large order to be placed so that kept them busy for a while getting it ready. They would giggle at my crazy order and when I wasn't playing they too ordered crazy combinations and laughed. We have a sun porch that has low windows, so we played through those windows. But if you do not have a window to play drive through then you have to create some sort of "peek through" area. You can do it with a small table with books stacked on the sides and two yardsticks across the books. Then top it with a bath towel to get a window look. Get creative! I bet most kids know the industry terms for this activity! So, make the playing fun by mimicking the real deal: **May I take your order? Do you want fries with that? Do you want a combo? Would you like to supersize that? What would you like on your sandwich? Etc.**

Favorite memory from my kids: "Making crazy food combinations to give to mom like a hamburger with an ice cream cone on top, and we gave it a funny name."

15. Hiking/Walking in the Woods or Park (physical)

Players: 2–6 is ideal
Age: 6 to teenage years
Items needed: Good boots or shoes and socks, water, cell phone, backpack, **first-aid kit.** Hoodies that zip up are the best because they can be removed and tied around the waist if you become hot. Sunscreen, sunglasses, and healthy snacks are good to have with you.
Season: Spring, summer, fall
Outdoors
Prep time: You may have to research and find a **park, wooded area, conservancy**, or **wetland trail** where you hike or walk.
Possible problems and tips: Insects, animals, tired kids, scared kids. A child who has never been in the woods may become very frightened because the scenery is so different.
Tips: Choose a **trail** or area that is appropriate for everyone's fitness level. Always check the weather before **hiking**. Tell someone where you will be. If you don't have a close park, look for anywhere that you can

walk outside safely with your kids. The idea is to get outside and walk as often as you can without looking at your phone! If you have a dog, walk the dog with your kid(s) daily.

Teach them about **nature, camping, navigation, maps, compasses, headlamps, sun protection, knives, fire, emergency shelter, tarps, nutrition,** and **hydration.**

Favorite memory from my kids: "Seeing water running in a real **stream** was cool!"

16. Hill Fun (physical)

Players: 1–3
Age: 3–5
Items needed: Broom or long rope and steep hill
Season: Summer
Outdoors
Prep time: Very little

For some reason, this is a blast for toddlers. My mom, my kid's grandma, actually started this and it is very simple. Just tell your toddlers to roll down the steep hill and give them help getting back up the hill with a broom handle. Teach them about **elevators, wells, garage doors, cranes, mechanical advantage, pulley systems, fixed pulleys, mobile pulleys, reducing force, exercise equipment pulleys, levers, lift, balance, stability,** and **anchoring.**

Possible problems: The adult holding the broom may get tired.

Favorite memory from my kids: "Grandma pulled us back up the hill with a broom!"

17. Homemade Dough

Players: 1–4
Age: 2–12
Items needed: See dough recipe below, plastic spoons and knives, cups, bowls, rolling pin, pans, cookie cutters, outdoor table(s), plastic to cover the table, garden hose or plastic empty soda bottle to fill with water, latex gloves (to prevent hands from getting stained from food coloring).
Season: Summer
Outdoors (recommended)
Prep time: 5 to 10 minutes (if you make the dough ahead of time then you will have less prep time but the dough is fun when it is warm)
Dough recipe:

2 cups flour, 1 cup salt, 4 tsp cream of tartar, 2 cups lukewarm water, 2 tbsp cooking oil, and food coloring if you want to color the dough. In a large pot, stir together the flour, salt, and cream of tartar. Add the water and oil. If you are only making one color of dough, add the food coloring now. Cook over medium heat stirring constantly until the dough has thickened and begins to form into a ball. Remove from heat and place inside a quart-size plastic bag or waxed paper to cool. If you are adding colors, divide the dough into balls for as many colors as you want, put the dough in the quart-size plastic bags, and add about 5 drops of food coloring. Close the bags and knead the dough as it is inside the bag; this will protect your hands from being stained. Add more color for more vibrant dough. After it is mixed you are ready to play. Store dough in plastic bags.

Possible problems: There is quite a lot of cleaning up after this activity. Only the brave will take on this activity indoors. You can make the dough ahead of time, or at least have the measured amounts ready **for your kids.** I highly recommend it for outdoor activity on a sunny day. The object is to make dough out of flour and water, then let your kids color the dough and make shapes and pretend food with it. This activity kept my kids busy for hours. Your kids can learn how two colors can make a third color such as red and blue make purple. They can learn how pizza dough is made by getting a proper consistency and using flour to take the "sticky" away. Teach them how to make **donut holes** and use **cookie cutters**. Teach them terms such as **kneading** the dough, **pressing** the dough into the pan, **color blending primary** and **secondary colors.**

Favorite memory from my kids: "We had fun making really pretty colors and the dough was so soft!"

18. Water Fun/Sprinkler

Players: 1 to a group
Age: 2–10
Items needed: Hats, sunscreen, T-shirts, a chair for parents, and a hose they can hold or a sprinkler for the kids to run through and play under if you have one. If you are in an urban environment, check for parks or a place that has sprinklers for kids to play in on hot summer days.
Season: Hot summer days
Outdoors
Prep time: a few minutes
Possible problems: Can be costly and some may frown upon water use; however, if you are concerned about water use you can fill a large tub or

plastic kid's pool and use a water can to sprinkle them. When they are done playing you can use the water for the garden, plants, or flowers.
Favorite memory from my kids: "Great fun! We loved this!"

19. Lemonade Stand

Players: 2–6
Age: 4–10
Items needed: For an official sale of lemonade: Lemonade stand or table, pitcher, water or lemonade, cups, cups or containers for money if selling the lemonade, paper and a marker for a sign to say Lemonade Stand, and change for clients. For non-official Lemonade Stand: fake credit cards (can save from mail offers), credit card swipe box (use your imagination — any kind of small box that you can pretend to slide a fake credit card through), food coloring, pitcher for water, spoons, flowers to put on top of drinks, cups, drink holders from fast-food restaurants.
Season: Summer
Outdoors
Prep time: Once you have the stand or table, just gather the cups, pitcher, and liquid.
I adore Lemonade Stands and always try to stop and purchase when I see kids doing this. These are future **entrepreneurs**! It is not hard to set up **a table and a sign** and gather all the items needed. It is good to have the stand near people or traffic but not too close. My kids did this a few times but mostly liked to play with the Lemonade Stand in the backyard by the pool where they could make crazy non-drinkable pretend concoctions by using water from the pool. Mud and water with sticks in it, grass and water, rocks and water, play dough and water, and food coloring and water. The Lemonade Stand brought hours and years of fun. I watched the brand-new Lemonade Stand that their grandfather made them age until it was pretty old, and they were still using it. It was a great gift and, in my opinion, well worth getting if you want your kids to have fun and be experimental with nature outside. If you don't have a pool, just fill up a bucket or pitcher of water for them to play with. A stand can be created out of cardboard as well. Teach them about **the seller, buyer, payment, cash, credit cards, bank card machine, merchant, purchase, tax, order**, **refund, profit, loss,** and **revenue**.
Possible problems: Most kids want to pour the lemonade and not buy it.
Favorite memory from my kids: "The best part was when mom gave us real money to play with! It always reminded me of my grandpa because

he made the lemonade stand and it was so cute, but after a while, the paint started to chip off."

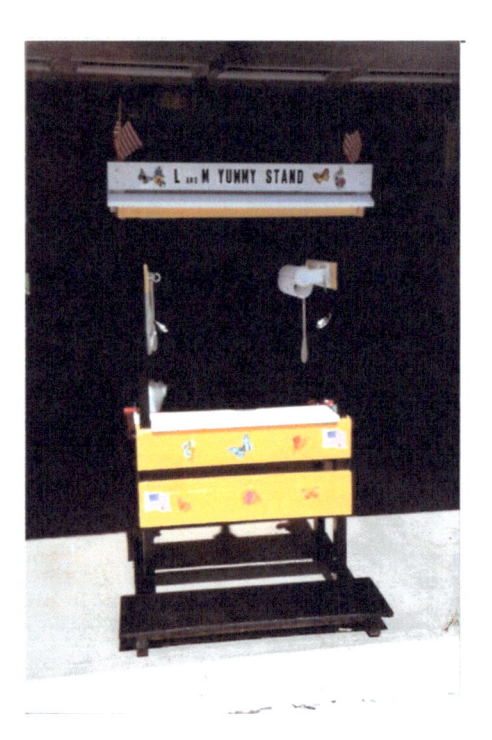

20. Living Room Gym /Obstacle Course (physical)

Players: 2–6
Age: 2–8
Items needed: A **stopwatch**, paper to make **start** and finish signs, a big space either a living room, basement or if you are outside, the possibilities are endless. Take advantage of your yard and be creative with **mapping out a course** and **stations**.
Season: Any
Indoors or outside
Prep time: 15 minutes to an hour. Depending on how intense your obstacle course is, it can take some time to set up.
Possible problems: Some kids may not want to follow the **rules** of the obstacle course.

Think of an obstacle course and what you can use that is already there in your landscape for your little **Ninja Warriors.** There are lots of suggestions online to help you create an at-home **obstacle course** outside. We mostly created them inside because there was enough to do outside in the summer that we didn't need an obstacle course. Indoor obstacle courses will be more challenging but there are tips online for them as well. Some ideas we used are **crawling** underneath a row of chairs, going under a string **(limbo style), jumping** from a spot into a further away **hula-hoop**, throwing a stuffed animal into a laundry basket, **tiptoeing** on a paper **balance beam** on the floor, hopping from pillow to pillow, and climbing over a sofa. Teach them about a **starting line, crab walking, bear walking, slithering like a snake, walking backward, walking sideways, dancing, walking with a book on your head, crawling, using bouncy balls or balloons, spinning, climbing, jumping jacks, burpees, push-ups, motor skills, and buckets, tongs or spoons, and balls.** The idea is to create a course suited to your child's age and interests. Try to make a course that takes some time to complete and when your child finishes, ask them if they think they can beat their time! **Favorite memory from my kids:** "We had to crawl under the dining room chairs and crawl through hula-hoops!"

21. Making Scenes—Toy Blending

Players: 1–4
Age: 5 plus
Items needed: A large table and toys that can make a city, town, or scene.
Season: Any
Indoors
Prep time: Just clear a large indoor table and help your kid(s) find some of their toys that can make a town, city, house, or scene. This is an open, creative, and imaginative game.

If you don't have a lot of toys, for example, you can make a scene out of some play dough. Make a small person or two, a bed, a chair, a TV, a dog, and then add to it. What else can you find that might fit into that scene? An upside-down plastic container could be a table or bathtub. Use a placemat for a carpet, 4 tall glasses with a dish towel over them can be a house/roof. If you have toys, such as a doll house and dolls or superheroes, use whatever you have to make a scene on the table. Toy houses, furniture, cars, farms, animals, etc. My daughters had one large doll house and we used materials to make different carpeting. They spent hours setting up different scenes in the doll house on my dining room table. We had a toy airport that they put on the opposite end of the table where their dolls could go to take a vacation. It was nice for them to be able to stand and decorate the scene instead of sitting on the floor! Smaller dollhouses can be far away to show distance and size correlation. Teach them about **communities, development, infrastructure, buildings, cities, counties, towns, suburbs, urban, rural, mountains, plateaus, valleys, country, neighborhoods, homes, porches, garages, barns,** and **sheds.**

Possible problem: Kids might not want to clean this up and put their toys away. They become proud of their creation and so you may have to leave it on your table for a few days or a week.

Favorite memory from my kids: "Telling mom about what we built."

22. Office

Players: 1–4
Age: 4–10
Items needed: Desk or table, telephone (real or pretend), paper, envelopes, stapler, pens, pencils, tape, garbage can, and any other office supplies such as calculator, stamps, ink pad, stickers, cardboard to make a "nameplate", books, pretend laptop, paper clips, high lighters, calendar, binder, notebook, ruler, erasers, folders, pencil sharpener, hole puncher, pretend fax machine, adding machine, radio, etc.
Season: Summer or winter
Indoors
Prep time: 10 to 15 minutes
Possible problems: This can get a little messy. Be sure to include a garbage can.

This activity lasted almost all day! My kids really enjoyed being "office workers". I set up two desks (a coffee table and another little end table) by a window and tried to mimic a **cubical**. I made nameplates with a title underneath for their **desks**. They helped place all of their office accessories. They were **stapling, cutting, gluing**, and pretending to talk on the phone. I gave them some ideas like how to pretend to **send a fax to a client**, place an order on the phone with a **supplier**, write a letter and put it in the **envelope**, make a call to get **approval for a purchase**, and how **to create an ad** for the **advertising department** or **marketing department**. I explained that their lunch hour would be at 12 noon, and they should get two 15-minute breaks. They really ran with this activity and kept very busy all day! Let your kids name the company where they work.

Teach them about **annual leave, management, co-worker, professional, conference room, time off, health benefits, paid leave, pension, retirement fund, 401K, vacation, email, partner,**
Favorite memory from my kids: "When mom set our desks up by the window so that we could have an office with a window!"

23. Old Clothes Design

Players: 1–3
Age: 6–16
Items needed: Old clothes that you can redesign by cutting—mostly T-shirts, good material scissors, style or clothing magazines for ideas, and markers to draw cut lines.
Season: Summer or winter
Indoors
Prep time: Time to find/collect old clothes and clothing magazines
Possible problems: This isn't the easiest activity, and the clothes may not turn out to be the redesign that was in mind, but it is a learning experience. This is an activity that my youngest daughter, to this day, loves and still redesigns clothing. Long sleeves can become short sleeves or no sleeves. Necklines can be altered. Holes and slits can be incorporated into the front, back, or sides of tops. Teach them about **fashion, tailoring, brands, patterns, seams, material, activewear, outerwear, sportswear, graphics, customize, pockets, collars, stitching, clothing lines,** and **embroidered, outfits.**
Favorite memory from my kids: "I was excited to do this because older kids did this to their clothes!"

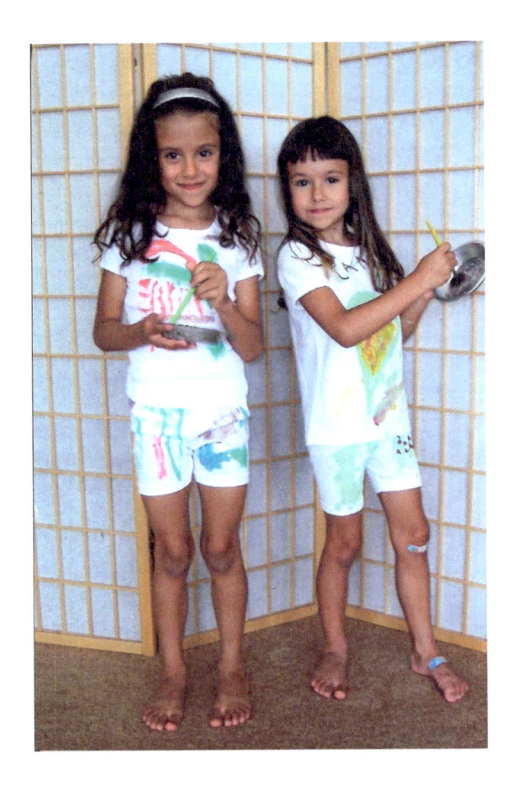

24. Painting White Clothes (can be added to the above activity)

Players: It depends on how many white pieces of clothing you have to paint

Age: 5–16

Items needed: White clothes, fabric paint, paintbrushes, bowls, newspaper or drop cloth to paint on.

Create ideas, find pictures or designs or logos for your kids to try to paint onto white clothing or free painting of whatever comes to their minds. Splatter painting, where you throw the paint onto clothing, is also fun but should be done outside. Use medium size brushes to dip into the paint and then flick at the clothing. Dripping paint onto clothes is also fun. Teach them about **graphics, custom, logo, design, pictures, words, art, slogans, original art, layout, template, images, font, silkscreen, printing, heat press,** and **heat transfers.**

Season: Summer or winter

Outdoor is ideal but indoors is optional

Prep time: 10 minutes once supplies are gathered

Possible problems: It can be messy.

Favorite memory from my kids: "Splatter painting clothes was really fun!"

25. Paper Dolls/People

Players: 1–6
Age: 4–10
Items Needed: Paper, scissors, art supplies, material scraps, yarn, plastic eyes.
Season: Summer or winter
Indoors
Prep time: 15 minutes to gather supplies
Possible problems: We never had any.

Cut out a doll/person from paper and then color them with markers, crayons, or colored pencils. Cut a string of dolls out or just one. (Search YouTube to see how to cut a string of dolls—little kids love pulling them apart). You can glue yarn on the dolls for hair, you can buy eyes from a craft store, and or use actual material to cut out clothing. Teach them about **crafts, decorating, yarn, material, glitter, glue, paste, cut, design, create, art, trim.**

Favorite memory from my kids: "Cutting them and decorating them was fun—pulling them apart was fun too. We did this again in school and called the doll Flat Stanley, and we had to mail it away to a friend or relative, and then they had to mail it back."

26. Pick a Question

Players: 1 to a group
Age: 4 and up
Items needed: Bowl or box and paper
Season: Summer or winter
Indoors
Prep time: ½ hour
Possible problems: None

It is just that unknown surprise of what they will pull out of the container that really makes the kids like playing this activity. At some point when your kids are sleeping or not around, get a piece of paper and write down as many **questions** that you think they could answer (age-appropriate). Once you write them all down on paper then you have to cut them out, fold each one in half, and put them into a box or bowl. Here are some ideas for questions: What is a baby cat called? What are three farm animals? What is a synonym for hot? Who discovered America?

What is your favorite movie? You can ask, where does the "setting" take place in their favorite movie or who are the main characters? You can ask math questions. I always liked to mix it up so that they didn't get bored. To catch them off guard, I would throw in a question like who is the cutest boy/girl in your class? You know how to make your kids laugh so throw in some crazy ones in between the educational ones! This can keep them busy for a long time depending on what kind of questions you ask and how many questions you can create. Wrong answers can require sit-ups, push-ups, jumping jacks, etc. Teach them about **quizzes, tests, questions, answers, correct, incorrect, math, history, science, English, social studies, trivia,** and **general knowledge.**

Favorite memory from my kids: "I used to get nervous!"

27. Pick To Draw

Players: 1 to group
Age: 3 and up
Items needed: Bowl or box and paper (using a mural—paper on the wall—makes this really fun)
Season: Summer or winter
Indoors/Outside
Prep time: 10 minutes to hang a mural, or if using paper, no prep time
Possible problems: None

Again, it is just that unknown surprise of what they will pull out of the container that really makes the kids enjoy playing this activity. At some point when your kids are sleeping or not around, get a piece of paper and write down as many ideas for things to draw as you can (age-appropriate). Once you write them all down on paper then you have to cut them out fold each one in half and put them into a box or bowl. Here are some ideas for what to draw: a snowman, cats, dogs, a house, birds, yourself, a tree, or a car. You can throw surprises in like your big toe! You know how to make your kids laugh so throw in some crazy ones! This can keep them busy for a long time! Teach them words like **drawing, art, picture, create, imagine, pen, pencil, crayon, marker, colored pencil, chalk, impromptu,** and **surprise.**

Favorite memory from my kids: "I liked when Mom would help us get started!"

28. Plays

Players: 3–10 is ideal
Age: 5–16
Items needed: A **script** with enough parts for the number of players that you have. This could take some time to find an age-appropriate play with just the right amount of parts. Gathering **props** and costumes for the play and creating a **setting** can all be done with your kids as part of the activity. You will need paper, scissors, and a marker to make **tickets** for grandparents, relatives, other parents, or friends. You can have a **presale** or sell tickets at the door. We always had our plays in the basement where we could leave the setting and all the props set up for a long period.
Season: Anytime
Outdoors or Indoors
Prep time: This could be an activity that you work on with your kids for a month or two days or a few times a week teaching them patience and preparation. Studying the script to learn the **lines** and having **dress rehearsals** will be fun. Teach them about **directors, producers, crew, cast, actors, actresses, lead roles, lighting, script, lines, sound**, and **rehearsing.**
Possible problems: Choosing who will be what **characters** may be tough if there is one popular hero or heroine.
Favorite memory from my kids: "We had light sabers and grandma and grandpa were invited to come and sit and watch our play."

29. Play-Doh® and Play-Doh® & Water

Players: 1–4
Age: 2–12
Items Needed: Play dough, water, plastic spoons and knives, cups, bowls, outdoor table(s), plastic to cover the table, and a garden hose or an empty plastic soda bottle to fill with water.
Season: Summer
Outdoors (recommended)
Prep time: 5 to 10 minutes
Possible problems: There is quite a lot of cleaning up after this activity. Play Dough is always fun but when your play dough gets a little hard and you are thinking about throwing it away, save it for a day in the sun outside. This is one of my kids' favorite things to do. Kids love **to mix, stir, pour**, and act like they are really creating something! I happen to be a clean fanatic and this is a hard one for me to endure, but seeing

their faces light up when they are making that squishy mess makes it all worth it. This activity can be very helpful in getting them a head start on understanding measurements which is usually in the third-grade math curriculum in the schools. They can learn the terms **change in consistency, liquid, mixture, paste, dilute, watery,** and **measures.** If you use **measuring cups** they can learn **1 cup,** ½ cup, ¼ cup, teaspoon, tablespoon, spatula, tongs, spoon, fork, knife, plate, bowl, and **cup.**
Favorite memory from my kids: "Making a big mess!"

30. Postal worker

Players: 1–4

Age: 4–8
Items needed: Unused mail offers and advertisements, a **backpack,** and shoe boxes to create **mailboxes.** Notepad and pen so kids can **sign** for their packages.
Season: Summer or winter
Indoor/Outdoor
Prep time: Saving enough unused mail to make the game fun can take some time (months). Have a certain box set aside to start collecting unused mail and once you have enough you can play. Create a mailbox for all kids from shoe boxes. Put their name or house number on the box. People used to have a flag on their mailbox that slid up and down and if you are creative enough, make a **flag** for the side of the mailbox that can go up to alert the **postal worker** when it contains mail.
Possible problems: When the unopened mail runs out the activity may become boring for some. Some may argue over who is the postal worker.
Kids love unopened mail, and you can teach them how to use a **letter opener** and put **stamps** and **return address stickers/labels** on new envelopes (mail often contains new envelopes). If you have some expired **visa cards** or fake cards that are included in **mail offers** they can pay for their mail to be **shipped** at the post office. Decorate a small box to look like a **bank card swipe machine** with a slice in it for the card. Create an area for each player to call their home where their mailbox will be. In corners, behind sofas, ends of hallways, bedrooms. Create a specific area for the **post office** where the **postal worker** will keep all the unopened mail. Teach them about **tracking numbers, ground shipping, 2-day priority, overnight shipping, insurance, Express, registered, certified, tracking your package, postal routes, zip codes hazardous items, toxic chemicals,** and **perishables.**

Favorite memory from my kids: "We used all the junk mail that mom had."

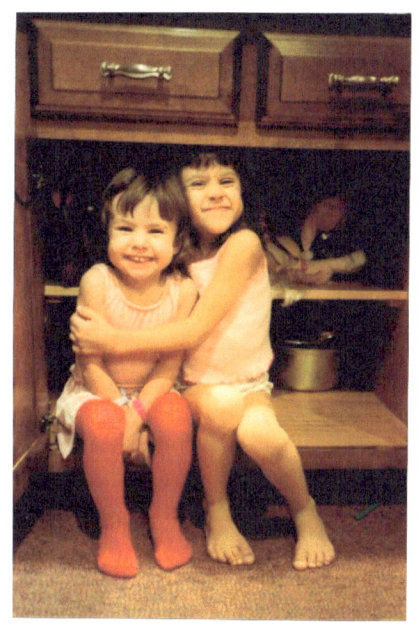

31. Pots & Pans Cupboard (another toddler favorite)

Players: 2
Age: 2–4
Items needed: Large cupboard or cabinet
Season: Summer or winter
Indoors
Prep time: Just remove all items out of the cabinet.
I have a large kitchen cabinet that I keep pots and pans in and it was great fun for my daughters when I emptied it and let them get inside. They would get in and out and in and out and shut the cabinet doors and giggle and get out and in for hours. A large box (large appliance) can serve the same purpose. Teach them about **storage, organization, cabinets, compartments, cupboards, units, space, self-storage, property managers, climate control,** and **rent money.**
Possible problems: None for my kids but always keep an eye on toddlers.
Favorite memory from my kids: "It was so fun and when we played hide-and-seek, that was always my sister's go-to place!" (The pots and pans cabinet.)

209

32. School

Players: At least 2
Age: 5–8
Items needed: Notebooks, pencils, crayons, markers, stapler, tape, scissors, construction paper, white paper, books, desk or table and **chair, flashcards.** Set up an area that mimics a **schoolroom,** chairs in a row, and a separate area for the teacher, **a bookshelf,** and **a blackboard or dry-erase board, etc.**
Season: Summer or winter
Indoors
Prep time: 20 minutes

Someone has to be the teacher and the others are the students. My kids and I literally spent countless hours playing school. Teach them about **class, teachers, students, classrooms, English, mathematics, spelling, science, history, social studies, visual arts, writing, lesson plans, pass, fail,** and **report cards.**
Possible problems: More than one wants to be the teacher.
Favorite memory from my kids: "Mom's name was always Lisa!"

33. School Bus

Players: 2–5
Age: 2–8
Items needed: dining-room chairs or kitchen chairs
Season: Any season
Indoors
Prep time: 5 or 10 minutes
Possible problems: We never had any problems other than your house is a little out of sorts.

This is one of the simplest activities for kids and seems to captivate the very young ones who may not be old enough to ride the school bus that their older siblings do. The concept is to create a bus with chairs. Definitely have your kids help you move the chairs if they are old enough. We have a sliding glass door, so we always put one row of chairs (each one in front of the other with about a foot in between) against the doors and those were window seats. We put another row of chairs next to those and then put the back of the couch up against the second row to sort of make a wall or side of the bus. I do not recommend moving the couch if you are unable to. My kids loved to play on the bus getting on and off. You can put a single chair upfront ahead of the others for the parent or a kid who might like to be the bus driver. Industry terms that you can introduce to your children are **bus stops, fares and bus passes, route change, detours, transit authority, HOV Lanes, park and ride lots, and rider rewards.**

Favorite memory from my kids: "When Mom drove the bus and went "chhhh" every time the bus stopped."

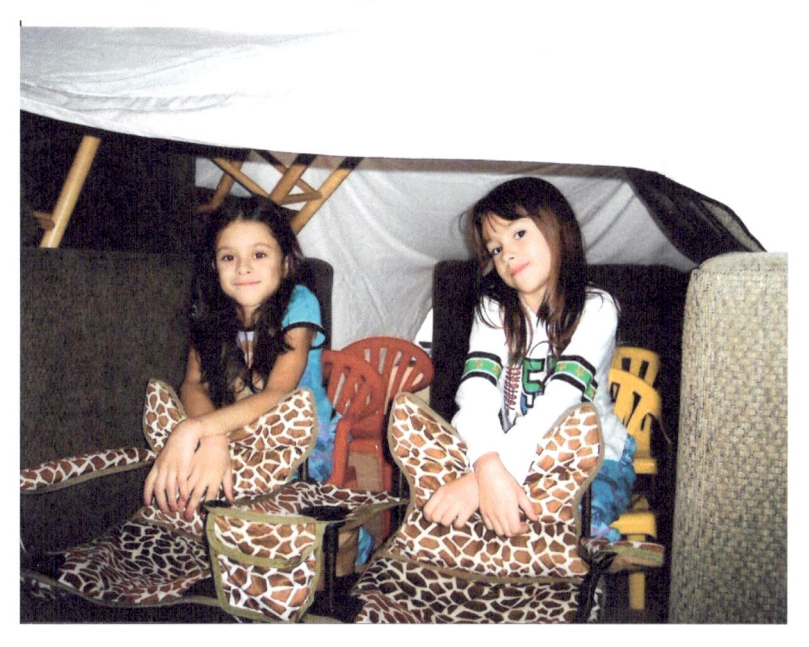

34. Sidewalk Chalk Town/ Bikes

For those who are unable to purchase a toy car; chalk and bikes are a fun alternative.

Age: 5 plus—must be able to ride a bike
Items needed: Bikes, chalk (preferably big chalk), and a cemented area that you can draw on and is large enough area you can ride your bikes through the roads that you create with chalk.
Season: Summer
Outdoors
Prep time: Create while you play but at least a half-hour to draw a road, arrows, stop signs, parking spaces, intersections, and store names.
Possible problems: You need a pretty big piece of cement or blacktop to draw roads. Drawing a road design on cement is difficult. It takes time and involves lots of bending over. Kids have to be patient while the paths are being drawn.

We were fortunate to have a fairly large driveway for this activity. If you do not have a large area of cement or blacktop you may be able to do this at your school on non-school days or at a church parking lot. We always started with the road. We drew a three-foot-wide path all around our driveway to ride bikes through. But if you don't have bikes you can walk through the paths. In one or two areas we drew **STOP** on the road. I asked my kids what kind of town they wanted to create (**city, suburban,** or **country**). Then we had to decide what kind of **businesses** we wanted to **construct**. We drew lakes with ducks to drive around so that our suburban town had **conservation**. We had a grocery store with parking spaces. Of course, we had to have an ice cream shop and a mall. While playing this activity we stumbled upon another activity when my youngest daughter did not want to stop for the stop signs. I became an **officer of the law,** pulled her over, and gave her a ticket. When she did not pay her ticket for her **traffic violation** on time we had to create a jail! My older daughter then became the **towing company** that **impounded** her **vehicle** and kept it in her **lot** until **jail time** was served! We also created a **school** in our **town** which was symbolized by a **flag**.

It is a lot of work but very fun and the chalk should last for a few days or even a week if there is no rain. Teach them about **driver safety, collision, driver distraction, driving lane, following distance, the field of vision, driver's license, license revocation, license suspension, safety belt, school zone, yield, tailgating, intersection, license plate, registration, inspection, yield, aggressive driver, speed limit, blind spot, braking distance, insurance.**

Favorite memory from my kids: "You actually get to drive through the chalk pathway. When Mom made the red tree the bank, and we pulled leaves off as money."

35. Sled Riding Fun (physical)

Players: 1 to a group
Age: 2–14
Items needed: SNOW! **Sleighs, saucers**, warm winter clothes, **ski wear**, hats, gloves, **snow boots**, shovels, lots of kids, and a few adults to help make a nice path.
Season: Winter
Outdoors
Prep time: Depends on how creative you want your **sleigh riding path** to be.

We live in Pittsburgh so normal winters are full of snow. We have a pretty steep hill in our backyard and when the kids were very young, we weren't sled riding. I asked my husband why, and he said he tried it but it didn't work. I realized that he grew up in the city and never had to make the sleigh-riding path. So, I went outside and started the path and I kept going down and down again until it was slick. He caught on and saw what it takes. Then he went crazy and in a few hours, we had a **bobsledding trail**. He brought out a shovel and covered a plastic summer toddler slide to be the **launch station**. He shoveled a foot-high wall along both sides of the path that had mounds and bends along with it. It was amazing, but then we realized all the running back up the hill was making my daughter's blood sugar low. I took a pitcher of orange juice outside that is how much of an impact sled riding has on blood sugar! We have a sun porch, and we put a heater in there and had hot chocolate for the kids—it was like a **ski resort chalet**! My father built a fire at the bottom of the hill. We had some music playing and 8 to 10 kids with the neighbors and mine. Teach them about **luge trails, skeletons, finish lines, riding conditions, ghost rides, snowmobiles, sleighs, trails,** and **curves.**

Possible problems: Too cold, too warm. This by far was one of my favorite activities with the kids!

Favorite memory from my kids: "A favorite! Like, sooo many memories! Dad took our plastic slide, covered it with snow, and made it a launchpad so we could go faster!"

36. Snow in the Sink (for colder climates)

Players: 1–2
Age: 4–12
Items needed: **A kitchen sink** (a double sink works well for two kids), **a large bowl for each child (to put snow in), food coloring, plastic clear cups, a large spoon, small spoons, measuring spoons, soup spoon, ice cream scoop, turkey basting device or droppers, cookie cutters, trays**. You may need plastic or a large towel on the floor in front of the sink if you have small children. I let my kids stand on chairs in front of the sink when they were very small so that they would be high enough to reach.
Season: Winter
Indoors/Need snow from outdoors
Prep time: 5 minutes

213

Possible problems: If you have children under 5 this can get a little messy. To avoid the food color staining anything, you can dilute it in little cups before you give it to the kids to play with.

Put a tray on the kitchen counter next to the sink and put the little cups on the tray. Fill the little cups with water and put several drops of food coloring in each to make one cup for each color. Fill the large bowl with snow and let the kids play. They can make different colors of snow and put it in larger clear cups, or they can make colored snowballs or snow cones. They can place a cookie cutter in the snow and then use a colored dropper to put the colored water inside the **cookie cutter** to color the snow, then lift and see if the shape is there. This is a great time to teach the kids **measurements**, use **tablespoons**, **teaspoons**, ½ teaspoons and ¼ teaspoons, **cups**, ¾ cups, ½ cups, and ¼ cups. If you have **pint**, **quart**, **gallon,** and **liter containers** you can introduce them as well.

Favorite memory from my kids: "It's like cooking! We would pretend that we were making snow cones."

37. Spa Day

Players: 2–4
Age: 6–12
Items needed: Footbath if you have one or you can use a big bowl, towels, lotion, nail polish and remover, headband to keep hair back, sofa, use your imagination!
Season: Any
Indoors
Prep time: Maybe 15 minutes to set up an area to mimic a spa in your home and gather spa items.
Possible problems: It can get messy with the foot soak and nail polish—best for older kids.

Have the kids take turns being the spa owner and the client. Teach them about **pedicures, manicures, massages, foot baths, lotions, nail polish, topcoats, French manicure, facials, relax, detox, complexion, skincare, pores, collagen, retinol, elastin, moisturizing.**

Favorite memory from my kids: "We used a foot bath and it bubbled over. There was one dark purple nail polish that was my favorite!"

38. Store/ Boutique — A Classic

Players: As many as you want
Age: 3–12
Items needed: A room, a play cash register or box for money, play money (can cut paper to make money), pretend credit cards, bags, and any items to sell such as clothes, books, toys, cars, and or trucks, paper to make "sale" signs and price tags, pens markers, crayons, receipts, etc.
Season: Summer or winter
Indoors
Prep time: 10 to 15 minutes.
Possible problems: There may be more than one child who wants to be the cashier!

Most kids love to play store. The basic idea here is to create an extraordinary store or boutique and that creative part seemed to always be the most fun for my kids. Getting them started should only take 10 to 15 minutes. I helped them once when they were very small by creating a checkout counter, a food section, a clothes section, a jewelry section, and a fitting room, and they played store for years after. When they became a little older I helped them make signs that said, **10% off**, **50% off**, **Red Tag Sale, Reduced**, **No Lay-Away**, **No Returns on Sale Items**, **Clearance Items**, and a **Fitting Room** sign. Playing store seemed to occupy them for hours and when their store was ready for the **grand opening** I always received an **invitation to attend** and see what they had created. Then, I had to purchase many items, many times and return them as well.

Favorite memory from my kids: "It was fun having our own store instead of going to a real one."

39. Swings & Squirt Bottle

Players: However many swings you have
Age: 6–12
Items needed: Must have a swing set or be able to go to a park or playground that has a swing, a powerful squirt bottle, and a chair for Mom or Dad.
Season: Summer
Outdoors
Prep time: You just need to fill up a water bottle, grab a chair, and go to the swing set with your kids.
Possible problems: None

For those that have kids, you must know how bored they can get in the hot summer. The end of July and early August can be tough. The kids are tired of the pool, you did the amusement park three times, and you took them to the park and parades. So now they are fighting with each other. Sometimes they can be downright mean and call each other names. So, I told my kids that if they want to let out their frustrations and be mean to someone then they could do this to me instead of their siblings or friends. I would take them to the swings outside and I would sit in a chair off to the side, and they were allowed to say silly things about me. The catch is if I would get my feelings hurt, I would get to squirt them. This sounds so silly but it really is fun. My girls ended up laughing so hard while they swung and made fun of Mom and of course they got soaked! You really need a big squirt bottle and one that you can put on "stream". It is a good way to teach them that comments can hurt feelings and to not take other people's comments so seriously. We honestly laughed so hard the entire time.

Favorite memory from my kids: "It was so fun we started out dry and always ended up soaking wet!!!!"

40. Tents/Tent Houses

Players: 1–6
Age: 2–10
Items Needed: If you have a tent of any kind or get creative with blankets. Kids LOVE being in tents or under a blanket and hidden! Once the tent is up or built ask the kids to decorate their tent house with their toys—**interior design and housewares.** My kids would bring stuffed animals into the tent and play phones and play laptops—**electronics.** We had a homemade tent so big one time that they were able to fit their play kitchen inside of it—**appliances.** They can add pillows and blankets—**bedding.** Ask them where their **mailbox** is and you can be the **postal worker** or **FedEx** and put unused mail in their mailbox. For the very creative, add a **doorbell, window,** or **interior lighting (we used battery camping lights)** and or exterior lighting to light up their home at night. The tents would stay up in our house for days! Outdoor tents are great as well, but we always had to worry about wind, rain, and animals if we left them standing. This was one of my kids' favorite activities!
Season: Any
Indoor or outdoor—weather permitting
Prep time: If you have a real tent the prep time is just setting up the tent, if you don't have a tent prep time can be pretty extensive. My

husband used to bring 2 × 4s (lumber) into our living room and or basement, and he would rearrange the furniture so it took a while sometimes.

Possible problems: Clean-up can be intense and I would strongly suggest asking the kids to help put things away! Tell them it is time to **relocate** and you are having an **estate sale** and everything must be sold. Also, if there is a problem between the kids inside the tent you won't be able to see what happened.

Favorite memory from my kids: "Either inside or out it was a blast, we had a Care Bear tent! Dad used to make us really cool tents in the living room!"

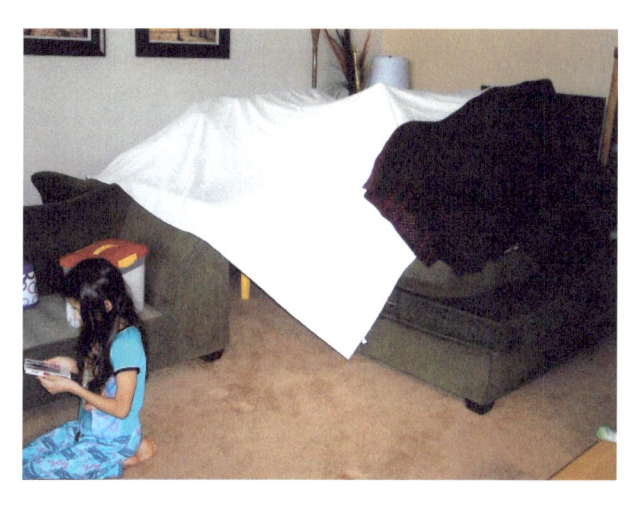

41. Tunnel—Cars/Balls/Kids

Players: 2–4
Age: 2–8
Items needed: Some kind of tunnel and a ball or toy car that can fit through the tunnel. Toy cars can be used if they can fit through the tunnel. Tunnels can be empty paper towel rolls taped together; or boxes with ends cut off and taped together. Sheets over two pieces of furniture or boxes can be used to make human tunnels for kids to crawl through.
Season: Summer or winter
Indoor/Outdoor
Prep time: Varies according to how intense your tunnel course is.
Possible problems: The Ball gets stuck due to bad course design.
Anything can be a tunnel as long as the ball disappears temporarily and then reappears and is still rolling. You can get creative and make

a ball/tunnel obstacle course with the ball going into a tunnel reappearing and then back into another tunnel and maybe landing in a bucket or bowl. Kids love disappearing items that then reappear! We did some crawling through human tunnels in our house. Teach them about **underpasses, overpasses, ramps, bridges, turnpikes, parkways, interstates, highways, Department of Transportation, detours, fuel, gasoline, fuel stations, bottlenecks, safety, miles, congestion, speed, roadside assistance, toll road, emergency response, merging traffic, police,** and **licenses.**

Favorite memory: "It was fun seeing the dog look for the ball to come out through the tunnel!"

42. Wall Mural Painting/ Drawing/ Coloring

Players: 2–4
Age: 5–16
Items needed: roll of paper to tape a long piece on the wall or fence or poster paper taped side by side to mimic a mural.
Season: Any
Outdoors or indoors
Prep time: 20 minutes to tape the paper on a fence outside or wall inside and gather the paints, brushes, and bowls.
Possible problems: Very fun activity and there should not be too many problems.

Kids draw all the time on paper but not often on huge murals. There is something about the size of the paper and standing while drawing that excites them. Teach them about **community murals as neighborhood art, graffiti, commercial murals, banners, live painting opportunity sites, art, artists, canvas, ceiling murals, Leonardo da Vinci, Diego Rivera, street art, paint, brushes, rags, sketching,** and **drop cloths.**

Favorite memory from my kids: "Making hand-prints was the most fun!"

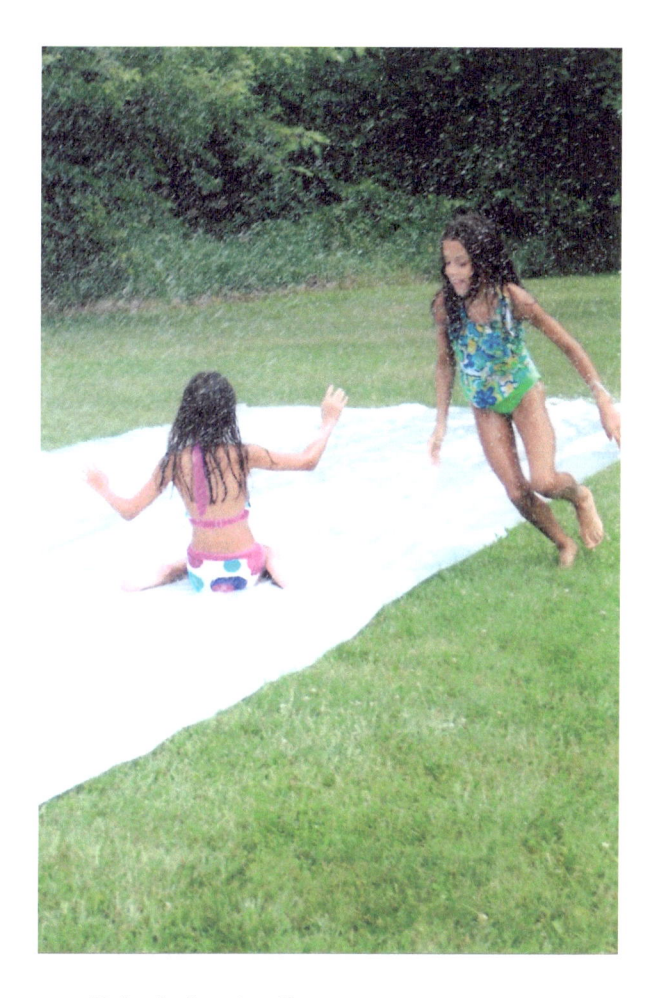

43. Water Slide (physical)

Players: 1 to a group
Age: 2–14
Items Needed: Sunscreen, **T-shirts**, **a big hill and a water slide**. You can purchase a water slide or use plastic from a home improvement store. **Dish soap** and **swimsuits**.
Season: Summer
Outdoors
Prep time: We had the intense bobsledding trail in the winter so it only made sense to have a water slide in the summer. So, we bought a 20-foot **water slide** but then used extra plastic from a home improvement store to add to the end and make the slide longer. We hooked the hose to the slide that we purchased and just made sure the slide stayed wet.

The kids would back up away from the slide, get a running start, and then dive and slide down the slide. They were used to going fast from the bobsledding path in the winter, so I added some dish soap to the slide which made them go faster!!! They were going so fast that at the end of the slide, they would continue on the grass past the plastic for another 5 feet making a muddy mess! To avoid using too much water, we shut the hose off and used a bucket and our pool water to once again wet the slide. Teach them about **water conservation, steep, climb, runs, the green light to go, taking turns, safety, thrill, slippery, lifeguard, water park,** and **theme parks.**
Possible problems: None!
Favorite memory from my kids: "When Mom added soap, and we went faster!"

Additional Play Suggestions That Require an Investment

44. Toy Car

I just want to add that this was a great investment. If you are near property where your kids can play I highly recommend purchasing the 12-volt little toy cars for them to drive around. My daughters drove their jeep for an unbelievable amount of hours for years. It was a two-seat jeep and when more than two kids were at our home, the others ran alongside the jeep. It provided great exercise as it kept them outside and walking, running, and playing. Even if you have to take them somewhere, like a park or a camp, to drive a toy car, I think it would be worth it. They started with a 6-volt and enjoyed it so much that they upgraded to a 12-volt and drove it for years! It is a great reason to go outside.
Age: 5 plus
Items needed: A toy battery or chargeable car and room to drive it.
Season: Outdoors
Prep time: Possible battery charge or transport to the area to drive.
Teach them about **driver safety, collision, driver distraction, driving lane, following distance, the field of vision, driver's license, license revocation, license suspension, safety belt, school zone, yield, tailgating, intersection, license plate, registration, inspection, yield, aggressive driver, speed limit, blind spot, braking distance, insurance.**
Possible problem: Not too many problems. Always keep an eye on kids when they are driving a toy car. Once another kid running behind the jeep pushed down on the back and the front end popped up. Let the kids know that a toy car is serious and no one should purposely wreck or hit another person.

45. Trampoline

The trampoline was another investment that I feel was worth the money and provided great exercise for the kids. They can be dangerous especially when there are too many kids on a trampoline and or a mix of little kids and bigger kids. With good supervision, a trampoline can be a great form of exercise.

A Life Skill Everyone Should Know

Swimming Pools

Swimming pools are great fun and exercise for kids whether you own one or you travel to one. Swimming lessons are really worth the investment due to the dangers of pools if children are unsupervised. Once your child can swim, take them to swim as often as you can. Remember, if you have no intentions of owning a pool or taking your child to a pool, swimming lessons are a skill that every human should know. If your child has had swimming lessons and already knows how to swim, go a step further and enroll them in lessons to become a lifeguard. I did this with a girlfriend in high school as an outside of school activity. I am forever grateful to my friend for suggesting this. Although lifeguard school was very challenging, it was a very rewarding experience and a skill I will always know.

Non-School Family Sports

Lots of parents have kids in sports at school but it is also good to teach kids that you can do a sport outside of school (like the Post-Organized Sports chapter in this book talks about) We chose snow skiing and, as a family, skied together while the kids were in grade school, middle school, and high school. There are many sports that you can do with your kids outside of the school environment. Here are some suggestions:

Archery, roller skating, ice skating, indoor climbing, yoga, trampoline parks, swimming, biking, snow skiing, cross-country skiing, water skiing, hiking, tennis, pool, soccer, croquet, volleyball, baseball, basketball, table tennis, surfing, lacrosse, ice hockey, softball, inline skating, futsal, water polo, skateboarding, ultimate frisbee, running, cycling, kayaking, white water rafting, canoeing, diving, paddle boarding, scuba diving, rowing, discus throwing, kickboxing, martial arts,

badminton, bowling, cricket, golf, kickball, polo, racquetball, rugby, darts, jogging, etc.

Now you have an idea about how to entertain your kids without using technology!!! These activities are just examples and ideas. You can now create your own list of fun activities to do with your kids.

Squeezing in More Daily Physical Activity and Setting an Example

I was on vacation with my family in Florida. I was with my two girls in the swimming pool playing volleyball. There was a woman on the side of the pool talking to another woman. She was telling her that because she was a schoolteacher she was unable to go to the gym and exercise because she worked all day and then came home and had to grade papers and then make the lesson plan for the next day. Exercise is tough to squeeze into your day. Remember, just a little can be a big help. My days are very busy as well but if you really want something, you can find a way. Just about everyone in America is watching TV. Make the TV room a little workout room. You can do yoga and floor stretching in front of the TV at night. In the morning, when my kids were little and liked to eat breakfast in the living room and watch TV, I kept my ankle weights and hand weights right beside the TV. I would work out my legs while my oldest daughter ate her breakfast, then when she would leave I would work out my arms and upper body while my youngest daughter ate her breakfast. If you spend a lot of time in the kitchen cooking, put on your ankle weights, use the kitchen counter as a bar, and do leg kicks to the back. You can transport small weights to any room that you are going to spend some time in. My 5- and 10-pound weights can be found all over the house! Treadmills are also a great investment for anyone who can't seem to get out to the gym. Whether I walk or run, it makes me feel good. The incline feature is great too for when you get bored with walking or running. I bought a stationary bike and I love it as well. Do I exercise every single day? No. I try to but of course, I miss a day or two sometimes. When I miss a week or two, that's when I start to feel edgy and tired. Exercise helps me alleviate stress and makes me feel good. Keep in mind that your kids are watching you and taking a mental note that you take care of your body and before long they may join you!

Conclusion – A Lifestyle Change

I sincerely hope that you have gained some insight from reading this book. The world of nutrition encompasses quite a lot and is ever-changing with new food items, new ingredients, new philosophies, and new recommendations, and it can be overwhelming to understand. I am not an expert, nor am I even certified in the nutrition profession. However, I was fortunate to be raised by a mom who was weight-conscious and a grandmother who was the same. Therefore, I had early nutrition awareness and dietary knowledge and was raised to eat healthy meals. I have watched the world of nutrition change and I have watched the impact it has had on the general population. In addition, having a toddler with Type 1 diabetes provided even deeper insight into how foods can affect our bodies. I have spent a lot of time researching nutritional information hoping to gain insight to help myself and my family and I believe I have. In this book, I am sharing selected relevant research to support some of my opinions. Good nutrition is a lifestyle for me and I have made studying about good nutrition also part of my lifestyle by continually reading and learning.

This book provides ideas and suggestions that worked for me and my personal circumstances. You may not agree with every aspect of this book, however, I hope that you can take away at least a few good tips and apply them to help you, your family, and your loved ones as they strive to achieve a healthy and nutritional lifestyle. Even if you do not lose weight, you may become healthier if you eat better.

About the Author

Jodi Velazquez was born and raised in Pittsburgh, Pennsylvania, and graduated from Robert Morris University with a bachelor's degree in marketing communications and an emphasis on writing. After graduating, Jodi left Pittsburgh to accompany her husband who accepted a job in Texas with the government. After multiple moves, and learning how stressful moving can be, Jodi self-published the "Slick Move Guide" to help others with relocation. The book is sold on Amazon and used by home builders, sports teams, moving companies, and the National Association of Realtors. In 2014, Jodi Velazquez was interviewed as an "Ultimate Expert" about relocation in Woman's World Magazine's April 24th Edition. The Slick Move Guide received the 2014 – 2015 TAZ Award for Business & Reference (Pittsburgh, PA author award). Over the years, Jodi has worked as an account executive, and she also was a TV Co-Host on Pittsburgh Community Television for eight years (2012 – 2020) on a show called "1st & 10 with Smokin' Jim and Jodi" where they interviewed sports and wellness professionals to enlighten the community. In 2020, Jodi was a content writer creating health and wellness articles for the Downtown Community Development Corporation - Common Thread, Pittsburgh, PA a bi-monthly newsletter. Her latest book, Know the Enemy: Preventing Weight Gain, Diabetes and Disease is a collection of 16 years of documenting her journey of helping her young daughter with diabetes management. Her daughter is now in her twenties. This memoir and self-help book details the discovery of healthy habits and good nutrition that paved the way for successful management which she incorporated into the entire family. Jodi worked with Atlas Elite Publishing Partners to produce and publish this book. She resides in Pittsburgh, PA with her husband and two daughters.

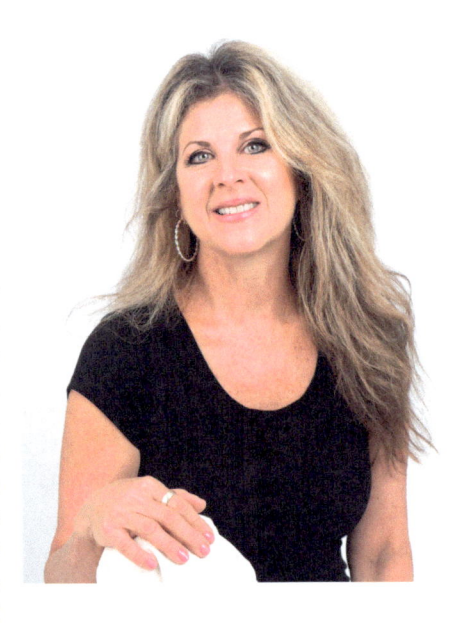

Interact with Jodi - Please check out her website, join her mailing list, watch her YouTube videos and subscribe!

Youtube Website